A Career
in
Speech Pathology

A Career in Speech Pathology

CHARLES VAN RIPER

Western Michigan University

PRENTICE-HALL, INC. *Englewood Cliffs, New Jersey 07632*

Van Riper, Charles Gage, 1905–
  A career in speech pathology.

    1. Speech therapy—Vocational guidance.   I.   Title.
[DNLM: 1. Health occupations.   2. Speech disorders.
WM21 V274c]
RC428.5.V35   616.8'55'0023   78-9678
ISBN 0-13-114769-2

© *1979 by* PRENTICE-HALL, INC., *Englewood Cliffs, N.J. 07632*

Printed in the United States of America
10 9 8 7 6 5 4 3 2 1

PRENTICE-HALL INTERNATIONAL, INC., *London*
PRENTICE-HALL OF AUSTRALIA PTY. LIMITED, *Sydney*
PRENTICE-HALL OF CANADA, LTD., *Toronto*
PRENTICE-HALL OF INDIA PRIVATE LIMITED, *New Delhi*
PRENTICE-HALL OF JAPAN, INC., *Tokyo*
PRENTICE-HALL OF SOUTHEAST ASIA PTE. LTD., *Singapore*
WHITEHALL BOOKS LIMITED, *Wellington, New Zealand*

contents

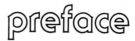
preface

The problem of teaching student speech pathologists clinical skills has always troubled the instructors who are responsible for their training. The basic information about the nature and the general management of the various speech disorders can be provided through texts and lectures but, as most of us would admit, these media are less successful in helping students with the clinical encounter. What we do is to give our students experiences under supervision in working with a very few, carefully selected clients or to have them observe experienced clinicians doing diagnostic examinations or demonstration therapy, either live or on videotape and film. No one is very happy about this situation; certainly the students are not. Most of them feel woefully unprepared to do the actual work of therapy (and they are), and most of their instructors can remember sharing these same feelings at the onset of their own practice. Must each new generation of students be doomed to stumble on the rocky road to competence making the same mistakes that we made? Or others uniquely their own? Is there any way that they could profit more from our experience?

In this book I have sought to design a very different kind of text, one that tries to teach some of the necessary clinical skills through metaphor and analogy, through the telling of tales, through anecdotes of actual casework and insightful commentary. Call it modeling or vicarious learning or what you will, students seem to learn a lot this way. The parable has taught more people how to respond to each other than all the texts on earth.

The stories in this text, though based on real people and real experiences, must be considered entirely fictional. I have often combined several clients into one; I have changed the kinds of speech disorders when possible; I have altered names, sex, and other personal characteristics to such an extent that identification would be too difficult. In the few instances where such camouflage was impossible, I have shown the tale to the client and received permission to record it.

I regret the host of perpendicular pronouns that dot these pages and I know that they will reveal more about my own frailty than that of my clients. So be it! I have learned much from my own mistakes and hopefully others will too. Finally, I hope that students will not gain the impression that all of their clients will show the dramatic problems of those pictured in this book. Certainly most of mine have not. But we learn most from those who challenge us most, and the individuals who people these pages were my teachers. May they also be yours!

CHARLES VAN RIPER
Western Michigan University

A Career
in
Speech Pathology

OUR CLIENTS

Clinical skills are hard to learn and even harder to teach. There are so many of them that one can spend a professional lifetime in their acquisition and still feel ill-equipped to do the job that must be done. Moreover, they cannot be mastered by memorizing a set of principles from a textbook any more than you can learn to swim by having another person tell you what to do. Facts and information can be acquired from books and stored in them, but not skills. One learns skills only by doing them, by trying them out, by making mistakes and correcting them, by blundering and improving. However, since it is also possible to learn through vicarious experience, i.e., by observing others perform these skills well or poorly, the beginning clinician need not greet the task of achieving some measure of clinical competence with dread. Indeed, that clinician can learn a lot by listening to older and more experienced workers tell their tales, even as the youth by a campfire ten thousand years ago heard the old cave men tell how they slew the saber-toothed tiger. Experience need not die out with each generation. It can be transmitted in many ways. So let us tell some tales.

Consider just the skills of interviewing or counseling. Certainly throughout our professional life we will need them in diagnosis and treatment. Many students approach their first diagnostic experience with forboding, and many of them ache after it is over when recalling their ineptitude. While it is impossible to prevent these feelings completely, perhaps some word pictures of some of our own interviewees will be helpful. We present them hesitantly, knowing well the dangers inherent in stereotypes, but you will surely meet some people who resemble them.

the overly verbal client

Some of your clients will respond to your first question by a torrent of miscellaneous and often irrelevant information that runs on and on. Unless you know how to react you may never get to that second question.

SPEECH PATHOLOGIST: Mrs. Jones, can you tell me something about how Willy's stuttering began?

MRS. JONES: Well, let me see. I know he was having trouble talking when he went to kindergarten over at the Miller Street School. He had to go on the bus, of course, and he traveled sometimes forty minutes which was a shame and I don't see why they can't do a better job of scheduling and I never could see any sense to busing anyway 'cause as my Uncle Toby always said if you spend your life on the road, how are you ever going to get things done. And my Uncle Toby was a bright man. And a lawyer. Well, not always a lawyer. He began first as a grocer but that never worked out. Got in one of those chains, you know the kind that got stores all over the city but I forget the name now. Maybe it was Scott's, but no, I think it was Harding's but anyway they had this place over west of town and. . . .

Some of these overly verbal clients can be interrupted by repeating your question swiftly at the precise moment the client finally has to inhale or die, but others who have mastered the art of quick shallow breathing will thwart you every time. Another strategy is to repeat something the person has just said and then to shift the conversation back to the topic. For example, you might have interrupted Mrs. Jones when she was talking about her Uncle Toby by interjecting, "You say your uncle was a very bright man. Is there some evidence that Willy inherited his brains? I'd like to hear more about Willy." If Mrs. Jones disregards your interruption, you calmly repeat it over and over, patiently not hurriedly, until she finally pays attention and responds appropriately. Two or three of these experiences are usually enough to achieve control of the situation and to keep the interview from becoming a disaster.

There are times, of course, when you are dealing with a person who at first talks continuously because he or she is obviously very anxious, as any dentist will tell you. Your wisest procedure in reacting to such an individual is simply to wait acceptingly until the compulsive flow of utterance ebbs, for any attempt to block it too soon merely increases the interviewee's anxiety. We remember a few such clients who made us feel like the peasant described by the Latin poet Horace: ". . . the peasant who sat by the river waiting for it to run by." But we waited.

When one of these flowing verbal fountains also speaks at an extremely fast rate, the clinician's problem increases in difficulty. There is always the tendency to start talking too fast yourself, a reaction which usually only speeds the speaker. One defense is to pretend to misunderstand, or in extremity, to throw up one's hands in despair and to wail, "I can't keep up with you. Please slow down!" Your client may think you're stupid but she will slow her speech temporarily, and then when she speeds up again, you can give the same arm raising as a silent signal. Some swift speakers will also slow down if you obviously relax, slump in your chair, look away or show some other evidence that you aren't listening. Some don't care whether you listen or not. *Tachylalia,* the technical word for excessive rapidity of speech, can present a real challenge to any clinician.

Certainly this is true when tachylalia accompanies *cluttering*—which it usually does. For years I failed with every clutterer who came my way, mainly because I did not have the essential clinical tool we now possess, a recording device so that such a client can hear himself. When I began to practice speech pathology in 1934, my entire equipment consisted of three tuning forks and a watch for audiometry, a throat mirror, and a box of tongue depressors. Over the years in sequence, I scrounged an old dictograph with a revolving wax cylinder, then an aluminum disc recorder so scratchy any speech inscribed could barely be understood, then a wire-recorder complete with in-house gremlins that created great tangles every time it was used, and finally the acetate disc and tape recorders currently in use. I should also mention that the microphones used with these instruments left much to be desired with respect to fidelity and so I failed with my clutterers.

The clutterer is a curious client in many ways. He often thinks and says that he is a stutterer, if indeed he recognizes that he has any abnormality of speech, and he rarely does. Clutterers seem absolutely oblivious to their own speech— which is why we need good recorders. They blurt and they spurt, but they don't hurt! They only hear their thoughts—which are usually pretty scrambled. Moreover, the cluttering disappears, as if by magic, as soon as the client speaks slowly, carefully and deliberately. He cannot bear to speak that way very long, however, for a normal rate of speech seems intolerably slow to him. Clutterers show repetitions, mainly of whole words and phrases rather than of sounds or syllables as in stuttering, and often their sounds and syllables are misarticulated and slurred in a most inconsistent fashion. Again, they can pronounce these perfectly and easily if asked to speak them carefully. If you could hear a tape of one of our clutterers, you wouldn't be able to understand him at all, for the rapid torrent of his utterance completely garbles his message.

One of these clutterers was Randy. Although he had done brilliantly at the university, majoring in business administration, he had been unable to hold any job for more than a week or two and had suffered many rejections from prospective employers who initially had been impressed by his written resumes. Most of them had been polite, if evasive, about their reasons for turning him down, but he finally met one who bluntly told him the real reason: "You talk too damned fast, and you stutter, and half the time nobody can figure out what the hell you're trying to say!" So Randy came to the clinic.

The diagnosis (of cluttering) was easy, but the interview was difficult. Not only was Randy frequently unintelligible because of his tachylalia and slurred articulation, he was also one of those verbal vultures who hover over your words and swoop down suddenly to take them out of your mouth and fly away. I would start to say something and he would finish it immediately—often incorrectly—in a compulsive flurry of extremely rapid and confused speech. It is difficult to indicate in print how he sounded. You really need to hear cluttering to appreciate it but perhaps this may give you a faint inkling—if you will read bis responses at 80 miles an hour.

CLINICIAN: Were the other members of your. . . .
RANDY: "My familyyesmymyyesmymothermy motherwas . . . well she-wasatensea tense . . . personson, personand . . . andshetalked, fashtveryfastlikeme. Allus talkedraplyverraply" (rapidly).

Randy spoke in spurts, in volleys, and the more aroused he became the more the cluttering manifested itself. When he really got going, he condensed longer words: *Kalamazoo* became *Kamzoo* and *superiority* turned into *spreeory*. Most of the blend sounds were slurred: *strawberry* became *srawbry*. But interspersed with these errors were occasional phrases or even whole sentences spoken perfectly, though very, very rapidly. I also found that when Randy was asked to read orally, at first his speech was much better, although he soon speeded up and again became almost unintelligible. He was asked to read the same passage backwards, word by word, and he did not make a single mistake, probably because it made him speak more slowly and carefully.

Since Randy occasionally referred to his cluttering as stuttering, and because there are some stutterers who clutter as well as some clutterers who stutter, I investigated this problem. His repetitions were of whole words and phrases. There were no prolongations or fixations, no difficulty in getting started, no tremors, no word fears or situation fears. No, he was a clutterer.

Only a general outline of the therapy can be provided. The basic objective, of course, was to get him to tolerate speaking more slowly and carefully. Our first task was to record large samples of his cluttered speech on both audio- and video-tape for later use. Then he was taught to shadow, to covertly echo almost simultaneously the speech of others so he could recognize that he was talking at a rate that far exceeded the norm. Next, Randy listened to the tape recordings he had made and tried to transcribe them on paper. When he discovered that he could not understand himself, he was unbelieving. It was just a bum recording, he said. So we had him converse with other persons while being recorded until he had to admit that they sounded very natural, even when his own speech was incomprehensible. We also used the delayed speech apparatus with a delay time set at two seconds. Randy had to hear the echo of each of his sentences completed before he could say anything else. This certainly slowed him down, but it also made him too frustrated, so instead he was taught to use verbal punctuation, saying 'comma' or 'period' (first aloud, then covertly). This too seemed to have little transfer. An operant program of contingent punishment and positive reinforcement was instituted which produced excellent speech in the therapy room, but again we could not design a transfer program that worked. The devil of it was that Randy could speak perfectly whenever he really set his mind to it. But once he said, "I can't stand talking that slow way. It's like walking through a quagmire. It isn't me talking; it's some zombie. And let me tell you something. Just having to listen to *you* drives me up the wall, you talk so slow, and so do other people. I'll never be able to talk that way!"

These moments are bad ones for the clinician—these times when you know well what the client must do, and yet know that he won't do it. By this time Randy had repeatedly heard himself talking very well on many tapes, and he had also heard himself rattling away unintelligibly. He knew what he had to do, and how he had to speak for the rest of his life, and he could not endure the prospect. As I desperately combed my mind, searching for an answer to the problem, I remembered what a physician friend had said about diabetics: "A lot of them just won't take their insulin until they've had a coma." How to get Randy to take his speech insulin? How to produce that coma? Some such vivid experience would have to be contrived to convince him that he would have to accept this new way of talking.

So we had an evaluation session, reviewing the entire course of therapy up to that time and also recalling his experiences in being fired from his job and being socially rejected because of his fast cluttered speech. I verbalized his hatred of having to monitor his speech so carefully. Then, with his permission, I put Randy in a therapy room where he could see himself on a videoscreen, and played that horrible videotape we had made during our very first session, turning up the volume. Sitting there beside him, even I could barely endure the sight and sound of all that monstrously garbled speech, but when the tape was finished I played it again—and again, until Randy, shaken to his roots, was obviously at the breaking point and ready to bolt from the room. Then he saw a brief videotape of the best conversational speech he had been able to achieve, an excellent sample, entirely normal, and I said to him, ''You have a choice, Randy.'' I then asked him to stay in the room by himself for another half hour, thinking. That something very important occurred during this session was soon apparent. Randy no longer was the passive resistant client he had been before. He worked hard on controlling his speech both in and out of the clinic and by the end of a month had acceptable speech in all situations. Randy also showed a marked personality change. He became less impulsive and fidgety. He became calmer, stronger, more organized, more direct—yes, more controlled.

But what had really happened? All clinicians know this disturbing question well. Was it merely the result of aversive conditioning, similar to that of putting an inveterate smoker in a smoke-filled room surrounded by cigarette butts until he cannot bear the smell or taste of a cigarette? Or had the traumatic confrontation of himself and his cluttering helped him realize that he would have to change both? Or what other explanation would be more plausible?

All I know is that a few years later, Randy, by then a very successful business man, told me that the most important half hour of his life had been the one he spent by himself *after* the video session.

When one of these overly verbal clients is encountered, learn to scan the speech for compulsivity—a feature which is difficult to define though easily recognizable. The more compulsively the person speaks, the stronger the emotional pressure behind the utterance tends to be. A description of an extreme and unusual case of logorrhea may help you remember this.

Mrs. Jones was a woman of forty years or so who had been referred to our speech clinic by her employer, the owner of a large restaurant. He said that she was the best cook he had ever had and would hate to lose her but that her speech problem was driving him and all his other help completely nuts and he was going to have to fire her.

When we examined the woman, no deviancy in articulation, voice, language or fluency could be discovered. Well, perhaps there was one in fluency. Mrs. Jones had *logorrhea*—the technical term for talking all the time. We heard her as she came up the stairs speaking in a torrent that never stopped for a second. In the waiting room she talked continuously to my secretary or to herself. The constant flow of her words persisted during our entire conference. No, it wasn't a conference but a marathon monologue, if that is the word for it. Moreover, she kept on speaking even when inhaling, a trick that most of us can master with enough practice though our inhaled phonation is usually weak. Not so with this woman. In and out, in and out, the chatter rattled on interminably. Most of the content seemed to be a sort of free association kind of utterance and it was also highly compulsive. I know she didn't hear a word I said. Completely unable to stop her even for an instant, I finally went out to see my secretary to escape the flood, and found the woman's husband there. (He had been parking the car.) "Sir," I said to him, "your wife doesn't have a speech problem; she has a psychiatric one. I suggest that you take her to a psychiatrist immediately." He seemed to have trouble hearing me. "I know," he finally answered. "I guess she's got to go back to the state hospital again." It was only then that I noticed he had plugs in both ears.

the non-responding client

In contrast, there are difficulties when trying to cope with the interviewee who responds laconically or not at all. Student clinicians have been known to climb the clinic walls after trying to talk with one of these clients. When each bit of information must be pumped out with immense effort, and the well repeatedly seems to run dry, the experience can be very frustrating.

STUDENT CLINICIAN: Mr. Smith, in your letter you said that your wife would bring your son. I do hope she's not ill.

MR. SMITH: Nope.

CLINICIAN: Can you tell me something about Bobby's speech at home as compared to school?

MR. SMITH: Nope.

CLINICIAN: How concerned are you or his mother about Bobby's speech?

MR. SMITH: Not much.

CLINICIAN: Mr. Smith, we need some information about the early development of Bobby's speech, whether he was slow in saying his first words, or saying sentences, and how hard it has been for other people to understand him. What could you tell me about these things?

MR. SMITH: (Long silence) Don't remember.

Most of these taciturn individuals begin to be more communicative as the interview proceeds and as the clinician reveals his competency. The important thing is to keep from feeling threatened by the silences and meager output. By reading the body language, one can usually determine if the person is being hostile, defensive or simply unconcerned. Then we verbalize our reflection and acceptance of these feelings, and continue by doing most of the talking ourselves. Often it is wise to talk about other clients with similar problems and how they were helped. Sooner or later, Mr. Smith will become interested enough to ask a question or to make a comment on some similarity, and once the conversational ice has been broken then you've got a chance. There are many other strategies that you will need to acquire for handling these individuals.

One of them is to escape from the therapy room. Some of our clients freeze up the moment they enter it. At best, it is not the ideal place to reveal oneself and you will find some persons who cannot be other than defensive when within its walls. Some of our most effective therapy ever done has been conducted outside the clinic and I'm sure that you will find the same need to escape its confines, certainly with some of the children you will serve.

So let me tell you about Tex, a very severe stutterer with long silent laryngeal blockings. A lean, hard-eyed professional gambler with a livid scar running from one eye to the corner of his mouth, he was one of the toughest clients we've ever dealt with. Tex just wouldn't talk—couldn't talk. At first we spent hour after hour in frustration and silence, during which he suffered the mute agonies of the damned—really suffered. I vainly tried all the approaches I could think of, even including writing out my questions and passing over a pad and pencil for his replies but all that came were crumbs of information. Finally, when in desperation I took Tex down to a bar and lubricated him thoroughly with bourbon, a totally different personality emerged: a very hilarious, free-wheeling, uninhibited soul, almost as fey as I am. After alcoholic lubrication, Tex stuttered very little and he talked a blue streak. Since he insisted I share his bottles, my memories of those sessions are not entirely clear but I did find out that once he had been a locomotive fireman and, because of his stuttering, had caused a bad train wreck in which several people, including some children, were killed. Tex had been unable to warn the engineer of the danger he had seen coming. Though this had happened some years before, every time he had another one of those long hard blocks he said he thought of that wreck and those dead children.

This information, this confession, was the turning point in therapy. Thereafter Tex was not so terribly alone. He had spoken the unspeakable, and since I had not flinched but had understood and accepted his agony, he found that he could talk to me even when sober. Nevertheless, this basic insight was not enough to free Tex from his stuttering. He still had to learn to modify those silent but severe strugglings in his throat rather than let them run their course. To him they seemed completely spasmodic and uncontrollable. It was difficult even to get Tex to throw himself into those hard blockings purposely so he could desensitize himself to their trauma and begin to get voluntary phonation. At the last instant he would always shy away from the experience.

My modeling of better ways of responding proved fruitless. Tex could not or would not follow my examples or directions. He would try but always fail. Although by this time he trusted me, he would not do what I asked him to do. At these moments of impasse, it is usually necessary to find additional forces to focus on the problem. We then need to marshall new and stronger reinforcements for the desired behaviors and, occasionally, appropriate penalties for the undesired ones.

Though it sounds a bit bizarre, you might be interested in how the problem was finally solved. I took Tex, the professional gambler, to an evening meeting of our Cultural Uplift Society, a small faculty group of men who played penny-ante poker with enthusiasm but without much skill. Amateurs of the first water! I told Tex we'd invented a new house rule just for him. Every time he put a chip in the pot, he had to say something, and every time he stuttered in his old hard way, we could each take a chip from his stack. Well, Tex just couldn't bear having neophytes and suckers take his gambling money away from him—which we did without mercy or loving kindness—so finally he did begin to modify his stuttering and skinned us thoroughly by the end of the evening! Another turning point, a breakthrough. He progressed rapidly from then on.

I still hear from Tex occasionally—usually about 2 A.M. He has just made another killing at gambling and he's feeling bourbon-gay. Says he hardly ever stutters any more, and he's certainly fluent enough. Too fluent for 2 A.M. The last time he called he insisted that I measure my feet. Tex was in Mexico somewhere and wanted to buy me a set of real cowboy boots. I told him I wore a size 82 and to go to bed in hell. He laughed. "OK, Doc, you old blue buzzard! Go back to bed yourself."

Student clinicians often feel pretty helpless when they meet a child client who will not talk to them. In most instances when this occurs, the child is responding negatively to the clinician's inappropriate behavior or to the demand characteristics of his or her language. We must remember that a direct question is always a demand and that any new relationship creates insecurity: "What right has this big stranger to give me commands?" And so the child clams up. Also, many beginning clinicians tend to come on too strong and too suddenly in the first encounter. The child must have the time to size you up, to make sure that you are no threat. He has to discover that you might be someone worth relating to. The experienced clinician provides the time and opportunity for this assessment; the inexperienced one may not.

STUDENT: (Rushing up to the child) Well, Jimmy, Jimmy! I'm so GLAD to see you! I'm going to be your new teacher. Won't that be nice? What a NICE boy you are! It's REALLY going to be fun working with you. Did you have fun at school today? Who's your teacher, Jimmy? How old are you, Jimmy? Do you have any brothers or sisters? Talk to me, Jimmy!

An older clinician would first talk quietly to Jimmy's mother, explaining what she planned to do and perhaps inviting her to come to the first session. She would probably begin by doing self-talk with the child, commenting on pictures or playthings she was showing and manipulating. "Let's see. We need a truck... Now where's the red truck?... Oh, there it is... And a bulldozer... No, that one's too big... Won't fit in the truck, I guess... Now let's take them over to the sandpile and..." During this solo play and talk, the clinician would not ask any questions, not even invite the child to participate. She would just play with the toys, talking quietly about what she was doing, perceiving or feeling. And when the child begins to play with some other toys, the clinician might occasionally do some parallel talking, occasionally commenting on what he is doing in the same quiet way. Then, moving slowly, she finds some way of having her toy and his toy first make contact and then later function jointly. (Her truck is steered to his barn.) A bit later, she may be asking questions but also answering them: "Oh, do you think we can get that truck out of the barn, Jimmy? Of course, we can. Guess you'll have to back it out though." And Jimmy will probably begin talking: "Yeah, no room to turn around inside." To watch such a clinician establishing a relationship with an insecure child is to appreciate the consummate skills and craftsmanship that our profession requires.

You may also occasionally meet the disorder of *voluntary mutism,* though it is relatively rare. Children with this problem just refuse to talk aloud. Some of them, the anxious ones, may communicate only by whispering; others, the manipulators, simply refuse to talk in any fashion and are truly mute. Voluntary mutism usually begins suddenly after a traumatic experience. Resembling school phobia in many ways, it should be treated as soon as possible because the longer it lasts, the more difficult it will be to regain the normal mode of communication.

I was once called in by a school principal to see a child who had suddenly stopped talking after his first day of school. The parents were sure that the kindergarten teacher was at fault and they were raising hell with everyone concerned. I interviewed the teacher, a lovely lady, warm and gentle, trying to discover what had happened and this is what she told me. Except for meeting her earlier that morning and talking with the boy in a group playing in the sandbox, the only other contact had occurred just after recess. She had asked Kenny to take his turn and to come up to the blackboard where he was to point to one of a number of pictures displayed there. She thought his picture was that of a ladder but couldn't be sure. Other children had preceded him in the task, and after they had named the picture she wrote the word under it. That was all. Except that when she had first asked him to come up to the board, he had refused, so she had gone down to his seat, and gently led him up front. "Many children are very shy the first day of school and so I try to help them see that everything's all right. When Kenny refused to point or to name the picture, I said, OK, some other time, and let him go back to his seat. He was crying but finally he stopped and I didn't think anything more about it. I swear that is all that happened. That was all!" I believed her, even if his parents did not, as they told me when I interviewed them.

The mother was especially suspicious and angry. "Something happened!" she insisted. "Kenny came home from school crying and he wouldn't or couldn't talk at all. And he hasn't said a word to us or to anyone else for three days. You can't tell me that teacher didn't do something bad to him. She ought to be fired."

So I saw the boy alone and it took two hours and all the skill I could muster before Kenny could whisper the explanation. While playing with the other children at recess, he had ripped the back seams of his pants, and the other kids, big and little, had teased him unmercifully about it. That's why he didn't want to go up in front of the class. And she made him go and he'd heard the kids giggling as he faced the blackboard. It was evident that Kenny had discovered that there was one thing no one could make you do—talk. Also, he had decided that if he didn't talk, he wouldn't have to go back to school, so he wouldn't talk at home either. Once we had this information, the Case of the Split Breeches was soon resolved.

I remember other children with voluntary mutism, but the one I recall best was a boy I didn't treat at all—one who was cured with a baseball bat. His name was Jonathan. Then in the fourth grade, he had not talked in school or on the school playground since first grade though it was said that he did talk a little at home. All the children in the first three grades of a school system had been screened (so that a new job for one of our graduates could be created) when the superintendent came in to observe. He told me about Jonathan and asked me to see the boy. First, some directions were written on some cards, and when he was asked to perform the activities, I noticed that he was sub-vocally articulating the words as he read them and that his lips and tongue moved appropriately as he figured out the harder words. His oral comprehension of my speech seemed to be excellent. There were no organic abnormalities and it was my impression that he was not hard of hearing. But he never said a word aloud or even in a whisper.

Jonathan had done well in school despite his handicap of muteness, the principal said in introducing us, so he was bright enough. Next, the boy was given the vertical board test of laterality in which he had to draw and write simultaneously with each hand on opposite sides of a board. To show him how to do it, I took his hands in mine and made them draw spirals. "Like this," I said, "Round, round round!" Distracted by the activity, Jonathan performed the circling and said aloud, "Round, round," then stopped and put his hand over his mouth with a sheepish look.

After the boy left, I told the principal that Jonathan could talk as well as we could, that the boy for one reason or another was just refusing to talk in school, and that he would just have to find some way to get him to do it. The screening proceeded.

A week later I received a letter from that principal. "Dear Sir," it said, "You were right about Jonathan. I've cured him. What I did was to take a baseball bat down to his fourth grade room, grab him by the collar, and drag him down to the boiler room, banging the bat against the wall at every corner. Then I raised the bat and yelled at him to say 'Round-round-round' just like you did, then to read aloud from a book, and then to say, 'I'm going to talk in school from now on.' And I raised the bat again. Well, he said everything aloud just perfectly so I took him back to his room and said to his teacher and all the other children, 'Jonathan's going to talk in school from now on, aren't you, Jonathan? Say yes!' Well he did, and he's been talking ever since. Thank you very much for your help. Very truly yours.'' May I say hastily that I do not recommend this kind of therapy for voluntary mutism even though it was effective for that particular child. Nevertheless, it is vitally important to find some way to break the wall of silence in these children, some way to get that first vocalized speech. How would you have helped Jonathan?

the weeping client

Many student clinicians, when confronted by a client who weeps consistently, make the mistake of being too sympathetic and trying to comfort or reassure the client when the tears drip down the nose and onto the office rug. But this only reinforces the behavior. The better response is just to hand the client a *full* box of tissues and to say, "Help yourself" in a casual, very calm voice. But you should also always add, "There's lots more." This phrase is what really stops the tears, for the thought of having to cry long enough to exhaust that first full box, and then other boxes as well, seems intolerable even to the most confirmed weeper. A colleague told me that he used a different tactic. He seated the weeper so she could not help but see herself in the large mirror behind his head. Once, he said, he even had to use what he had said to his wife when she began to use her tears to control him: "My God, you look ugly when you cry!" Sounded too brutal for my taste but then I did not know that client nor, for that matter, my colleague's wife.

This colleague was also an amateur ornithologist and he called such a client a Red-eyed Weeper. He said this bird could be identified not only by the color of its eyes but also by its drooping, bedraggled tail feathers and by its characteristic song of "Poor me! Poor little me." He added that its habitat was the deep swamp where it constantly indulged itself in the curious habit of wallowing in mud or its own excrement. He said he didn't like Red-eyed Weepers.

I must confess that I share some of that dislike and that it probably stems from the fact that in my youth, I myself did a lot of bathing in self-pity because of my severe stuttering. When one dislikes a client it is almost always possible to identify certain behaviors or features that point to one's own weaknesses. We reject in others that which we dislike in ourselves. Anyway, all of us need to recognize our biases and keep them from spoiling the clinical relationship. Sometimes it is very difficult to be sure that your clinical decisions are not being warped by your personal needs, as the following anecdote will illustrate. I think I did the right thing, but if you disagree, what would you have done differently?

The first time Phyllis entered my office she was weeping copiously—weeping for joy, she said. At last she had come to the Master, to the Fount. At last she had found the man who could cure the stuttering that had cursed her entire life. She ticked off all the speech clinics she had attended and all the numerous therapists who had *not* helped her. I could see her watching me through wet eyelashes.

"Oh, oh," I said to myself. "Another poor devil of an Ancient Mariner, complete with albatross, wandering the wastelands, hunting for yet another ear to fill with The Sad Story." All clinicians sooner or later will be victimized by such clients. They come to us pleading for help but they won't do the work of therapy. They drink deeply of our energy and our small cup of time. They blandish us with phony appreciation and devotion. Some of them are very ingenious as they spin their webs to embroil us in their lives and justify their suffering.

Not Phyllis. Her act was so phony it was almost unbelievable. Every session was a wet one. Every few minutes her lower lip would tremble and the tears would cascade down her cheeks. Phyllis didn't even stutter very much, but when she did it was with a whimper. And with the neurotic's brave little bittersweet smile! "Lord," I thought, "what a way to have to go through life! Wandering and searching and telling her sad tale."

It soon became evident that Phyllis had little interest in doing any real work on her speech problem. She just wanted my ear for a toilet. After the first three sessions I felt I was listening to a soap opera, a tear-jerker. The rejecting mother. The beautiful sister who had done so well. Her own tragic love life! The many therapists who had failed to help her, who had betrayed her! And on and on and on, all of it sobbed in the utmost detail and with a tear for every comma and period. It also sounded well rehearsed.

I fought down my growing irritation. How could I help this poor driven creature? What could I do to break the evil spell? Perhaps, after the weeping well had run dry, Phyllis might be able to grapple with her problem. No, then she'd quit and go elsewhere to tell her tale again. I cautioned myself to remember my own bias against self-pity.

But in our ninth session I did not let her speak a word. "Phyllis," I said, "you are a female Ancient Mariner doomed to wander forever, doomed to tell your sad tale forever unless you make a drastic change." Then, almost brutally, I described the dynamics of her self-defeating behaviors and showed where they would probably lead. With a verbal scalpel I flayed off all the pretense and laid her problem bare. "Enough of this self-pity on which you feed! God knows more than enough!" I said. And then I told her to get out, that our therapy was terminated.

Follow-up was, of course, impossible, but seven years later I found her name in our ASHA Directory. If by chance she reads this book perhaps she will write me to tell me whether the albatross still hangs around her neck. Is it ever kinder to be unkind? All I know is that in that last session I never saw a single tear.

Now of course the shedding of an occasional tear or more by a client should be accepted completely, and at times even encouraged as a legitimate means of relief. We all need safety valves. It is the client who seeks to exploit the clinician and to control him with her wet weaponry that must be treated differently. When the tears serve as a defense against having to face what must be confronted, when they are clearly manipulative, a too sympathetic response on the part of the clinician is inappropriate. But there are other times when it is good for the client to weep.

I remember well, for example, the desperate father who sobbed as he told us of his son who had a cleft palate. "I love my son, but for seven years now I've worked two jobs, day and night, to earn the thousands and thousands of dollars I've had to pour into his sad little mouth, and now they tell me he has to have orthodontia! I'm at the end of my rope. I can't pay those bills. I can't work three jobs. And, poor little kid, he still can't talk right." It's hard to see a strong man weep hopelessly.

the hostile client

Now let me speak directly about the difficulties we encounter when we must work with or interview a client who is hostile. Student clinicians tend to find the experience of being hated very disturbing; the old pros take it in their stride. They know that they are not there in the therapy room to be loved but to serve. Indeed, they would far rather have a hostile client than an apathetic one, for they know that hate contains the energy and strength that can be redirected toward the solution of the problem. Moreover, over the years these older clinicians have also developed a certain amount of scar tissue.

The body language of an openly hostile client is easy to read even before he speaks. The jaw is thrust forward. The lips are tight or the teeth are as clenched as his fists. The posture is rigid. The eyes are narrowed and the eyebrows are lowered as were those of Tam O'Shanter's wife in the poem by Robert Burns:

> "Gathering her brows like gathering storm,
> Nursing her wrath to keep it warm."

When most of these signs appear, the experienced clinician knows that Mt. Vesuvius is about to erupt. But she does not flinch. She keeps her cool and tries hard to understand the nature and causes of the pressures that provoke the lava flow. Or at least she tries to stay cool. Emotional lava can be very hot, and most of us have been burned a bit at one time or another. So be it! Unto their needs!

One common error made by beginners is to attempt to ignore the client's demonstrations or verbalizations of hostility, to pretend that no anger has been shown. This is unwise unless you want to increase the person's fury in the interest of further catharsis. In most instances, the better way is simply to verbalize the client's rage, showing him that you understand its intensity and accept his need to express it. You will find that after the thunder and lightning have passed the air will be clearer. If you feel too vulnerable to the arrows of your

18

client's hate, put on the only armor we have available—the armor of the clinician's interest and dedication. No one can change a client if he's full to the brim with fury. The client can only listen to the yelling of his glands, so he won't be able to hear what you say. He can't be reasonable until the pressure is relieved. So you'd better recognize that one of your many clinical roles will be that of a safety valve.

Here is the transcript of an interview with a very verbal, very angry classroom teacher. I have deliberately omitted all of my own responses. After each of her volleys, try to guess what might have been said, or try to formulate your own appropriate response.

TEACHER: "These speech therapists, or speech correctionists, or whatever you want to call them, sure *burn* me up! And I think it's time somebody said what all of us classroom teachers are thinking about them. I think they're a bunch of frauds and here's why: first of all they don't teach or act like teachers! I've looked through the window of the speech room more than once and what do I see? The children, even fourth graders, are playing games, horsing and fooling around, making faces, laughing, and the teacher is right in there fooling around with them in the same way. Darn little discipline so far as I can see, and even less speech. How do they get away with it? I think it's about time someone called their bluff . . ."

CLINICIAN: (How do you think I responded?)

TEACHER: "Oh, don't give me that stuff. Maybe there are some speech correctionists who know what they're doing, but you ought to see some of these extra fancy special speech therapists we've had in our building in the last few years. They act as if they are God's gift to the lisper. They've come to save the human race from baby talk. How come they have to pretend they're so professional? Why don't they wear a white coat like the nurse? To hear them talk, you'd think they were a branch of the medical profession. They're paid by the school board same as I am. But do they do hall duty? Or collect milk money? Or help at recess? Or mark papers? Or put on ovrshoes? Not milady speech therapist, not she! She's right there at coffee break time though, and she smokes a long cigarette. Never saw one of them yet at a PTA meeting and seldom at a teacher's meeting. *Are* they teachers or aren't they? If you ask me, they're too darned independent. It sure burns me up to see one of them walk out the front door of our school in the middle of the morning and get into her car. Boy, what a racket! Mebbe I should quit and get my master's in speech correction and get some of that gravy."

CLINICIAN: . . .

TEACHER: "Oh, yes, yes, yes, yes, yes. You sound awful good, but mister, you're not convincing. I've known these speech correctionists in the corridors and just fresh from the ivory tower. The trouble with speech correction is that it doesn't correct! There's a little girl in my room now . . . I teach third grade . . . and she's had speech correction for three years and she still talks out of her nose. And I've had kids who stuttered who got worse right away when they went to the speech correctionist. Oh, I've seen some of them learn to speak better but they probably are just outgrowing it. I bet they'd do just as well if they didn't have any speech help. I've seen children do it before. How come they take credit for maturation? And another thing . . . you ought to see how many times they send me a note and say that Jimmy or Johnny is now able to say his sounds all right and that he is being dismissed. Why you ought to hear 'em in class recitation. All kinds of mistakes and lousy speech still. It's a racket, I tell you. They don't do what they're supposed to do. And I hear they get a differential in salary. What a deal!"

CLINICIAN: . . .

TEACHER: "So you say . . . So you say . . . Now let me tell you something else. These speech correctionists are always asking for my help—for *my* cooperation, please, in seeing that Sally remembers to keep her dirty little teeth closed when she says her S sounds or to wait patiently while Willie stutters without interrupting him. And can I tell her how he is doing in school lately? And from what kind of a home does Bob come? Why the devil doesn't she find out herself? And why should I help her when she doesn't help me? Cooperation should work both ways. Wait for little Willie, hey? How long? Oh, Lord, how long shall we wait for Willie? All Willie has to do is to get stuck on one word and the whole class goes to pot. *She's* the one they pay to do the speech correction. Why should I do her job for her?

CLINICIAN: . . .

It is not too difficult to deal appropriately with an angry teacher or parent in a one-shot interview, but your professional skills will be really tested when you must do long term therapy with a hostile client. There have been many times when I dreaded having once again to endure the daily attack which I knew was coming. And there have been times after such a hate session when I felt both drained and smeared, and, I must confess, even resentful. Clinicians must learn to accept and forgive their own weaknesses as well as those of their clients, but I don't like myself when I sense that resentment. What I've learned to do when those feelings come is to hunt for a moment to escape so I can cleanse myself.

There are many reasons for hostility, all of them clinically legitimate. Some of our clients are full of hate because they themselves have been hated and hurt by those who should have loved them. In others, the anger seems to be a protective mechanism, a way of saying, "Stay away from me, dammit! I've learned not to trust anyone." Sometimes the hostility is merely a conversion of anxiety that has become intolerable. More rarely, the client attacks you because he wants you in turn to whip him as penance for some hidden guilt. But the most frequent source of the hostility that I have found in my own practice has been frustration.

It is difficult for normal speakers to appreciate the intensity of the frustration experienced by persons with severe speech disorders. We have watched little children bang their heads against the wall or spit on their mothers when they tried in vain to make themselves understood. We remember Ivan the Terrible, an unintelligible hyperactive boy, who would swarm up and bite his grandmother on the nose when she couldn't make out what he was saying. We have watched the catastrophic rage sweep over a person with aphasia when he could not find the words he needed or when jargon came out of his mouth. As for stutterers, there are a hundred tales of how their intermittently blocked speech resulted in a hundred forms of aggression.

All clinicians sooner or later come to recognize that frustration leads to aggression, that aggression can be turned outward in the form of attacking others, or turned inward to become some form of self-hatred. Also, they know that it is better to have hatred come out than to stay inside the soul sack. Anger is a corrosive acid that eats its container, and it can burn the clinician, too, if it is not handled carefully.

Of all the ways to end one's days, one of the worst is to have a severe stroke resulting in a profound aphasia. In my practice I've had to work with many of these patients, trying desperately to help them regain the ability to speak or read or write or even to comprehend what others are saying to them. The physicians speak of a stroke as a "cerebral insult" but the experience is much more than that. In a few terrible moments, the person loses his identity and his membership in the human race, for you have to be able to send and receive messages to belong to that race. He does not know or cannot speak his name; he cannot count or tell time or write his name on a check. He may not recognize his wife. He may open his mouth to speak and gibberish comes out of it. One half of his body may be paralyzed. It is catastrophe.

But let me tell you about one of them. After I had addressed a group of nurses to provide them with information about various forms of speech pathology, one of them came up afterward and told me about a forty-year-old man with aphasia who had been cared for in a private nursing home for three years after his wife abandoned him. He had never had a visitor in all that time. "His name is Harry," she said, "and I think he understands what others say to him but all he ever says is 'Bumadee.' He says it over and over again and it sure sounds like he's trying to tell me something. He can't write but will point to something he wants with his good arm. The doctor says nothing can be done but I wish you'd go down to see him. The old gal who runs the place is a bitch and doesn't want visitors in her dump but I'll make the arrangements if you can manage it."

I managed. The nursing home was indeed a dump, a firetrap of an old frame building. When I stated the purpose of my visit, the proprietor reluctantly let me in. She was obese and wheezed as she led me upstairs. "There's two in this here room, Joe and Harry. Harry's the one you come to see—though I don't know what you think you can do for him. He's sho . A dummy. Can't talk nothing but nonsense. I figure he'll kick the bucket ar y time now. Hopeless. I'll put him in the wheelchair for you." Somehow, she wrestled the man into it, cursing him for not cooperating. Then pantingly she lumbered off. Harry and I eyed each other.

The first confrontation with a severe aphasic patient must be handled with care. I pointed to myself and said "Speech doctor" several times, slowly and with plenty of pause between each utterance. Finally his face lit up and he pointed to his mouth and shook his head sidewise and began to cry and laugh. "Umadee bumadee, um, um, bum, umadee." A torrent of this utterance poured out of the man and he became so excited he almost fell out of his wheelchair. I waited calmly until the emotion was spent, then pointed to him and said "Harry?" Again the paroxysm of emotion and gibberish and again the negative shaking of the head. "Ah," I thought, "he's got his gestures of affirmation and rejection reversed. He nods sideways for yes." This was checked in several ways and it was true. The Bulgarians nod in the same way. I must remember to consider Harry a Bulgarian. His visual reception was tested. He could read nothing aloud or silently. He was unable even to match the singly printed word "shoe" with either a picture of a shoe or the actual object on my foot. That avenue was evidently closed. I explored his auditory comprehension. It was much better. If I spoke very slowly and simply and gave him plenty of time to decode, he could usually point to any object I mentioned and to follow simple commands. Good, we might be able to use this facility. I tried having him write words from dictation. He took the pencil awkwardly in his unparalyzed hand, the left one, but only made squiggles on the paper before he began to cry again. I pulled out my pipe and lit it.

Harry became excited and tried to tell me something. "Umadee, uh, uh, oh, dum, dumadee, oh." Consumed with utter frustration, he dropped and sighed and shook his head up and down. I waited. Finally he roused himself, puckered his lips and gasped three times. I did not understand. With his good hand he propelled the chair over to me and reached for my pipe, made motions as if to put it in his mouth, then nodded up and down when I asked him if he wanted me to bring him a pipe and tobacco. He again nodded his head vertically and I remembered that he was trying to say no. I must have looked a bit confused for Harry then patted my hand reassuringly. As he did so, again that light illuminated his face. With his forefinger, he first pointed to his mouth and then tapped my ear three times. "Ah!" I understood. He was tapping out the syllables for "cig-a-rette." I took his finger and tapped my mouth and said the word over and over again, a syllable with each tap. Then I used it to tap his own mouth and out of it came a garbled but distinguishable word resembling cigarette and certainly completely different from "umadee." I responded. "OK, Harry . . . Bring you cigarette . . . cigarette (I tapped his lips lightly)... Bring you cigarette... Go now... Come back soon... Bring Harry cigarette.'' Weeping and smiling, he took my hand and put it on his wet eyes and then on his mouth. It was hard to leave when I saw fear in his face that I might not return.

Return I did... almost every day for many months. Harry had two wonderful years before he died. With the help of my students—who also visited him several hours each day and even brought him up to the university clinic at times to speak before my classes—he regained a substantial amount of speech, though he never learned to read and write with any facility. Some of my colleagues wondered how I could spend so much of my own small cup of time on a person so handicapped and so likely to pass away at any time. I told them that Harry was my teacher, that I had learned much from him, and that anyway all of us were similarly en route to eventual death. The thing was to live well meanwhile. Harry did.

Therapy was very difficult at first and, even later, Harry would seem to reach a plateau and fail to make further growth. There were many problems. Let me tell you about just one of them. Many aphasic patients show a loss of emotional control. They experience profound emotional storms. They over-laugh and cannot stop; they weep and continue weeping; they rage. Physiologists have found the same behavior in decorticated cats. The slightest stimulus will set off a paroxysm of hissing, scratching and biting that keeps going until the cat falls exhausted to the floor of the cage. Our human cortex, like the cat's, has many functions and one of them is to inhibit such emotional display. The aphasic, whose cortex has also been injured, tends to respond in much the same way. You can probably imagine how this hairtriggerness interferes with therapy. Often we have to work very hard to reestablish these inhibitor controls so our work can proceed.

Harry showed this emotional lability in extreme degree but gradually he responded to some operant conditioning and learned to calm himself, first when I gave a finger signal and later when he gave it himself. I was, therefore, a bit surprised when one day I found him screaming and crying and thrashing around in the bed. All he could say again was "umadee umadee." My signals did not help. He did not even seem able to listen to me. He kept trying to tell me something but he was wild. I finally went over to the bed, straddled him, took his head in my hands and held him by main force until his struggles subsided and he became silent. Then I drove him hard, insisting upon his doing what I asked, shaping and manipulating his mouth, pressing on his chest so he would remember again that he had to speak on exhaled rather than inhaled air. When he occasionally began to become excited, I gave him hell and insisted that he calm down and do what I demanded. Surprisingly, Harry made great gains that day, spoke in sentences for the first time, and even called the nurse and asked for a drink of water at the end of the session.

As I left, completely exhausted, the old slatternly battle-axe who owned the nursing home asked me how I got along with Harry. I told her I'd had a hell of a time, that he was wild as a hoot owl, but in spite of it we'd made some progress. She grinned evilly as I went out the door and said, "I probably should have told you that Joe, the other guy behind the screen in Harry's room, kicked the bucket and died just before you came in. He's still there in the other bed." That was what Harry had tried to tell me! I still feel badly about that session, though I shouldn't.

Here is another case-illustration of self-aggression resulting from extreme frustration.

Mr. G. was a laryngectomee. Before the surgery that removed his entire larynx because of the cancer that threatened his life, he had been a very successful trial lawyer. His wife described him as being impatient, very aggressive, and prone to displays of temper. This was not the picture he presented when I first saw him. Instead he was in the lowest part of a depression so deep that he sat immobile, with glazed eyes, completely detached. Nothing I did or said seemed to pass the barriers, so I told his wife he was not ready for therapy, that many laryngectomees reacted that way when they found that they were completely mute, but that usually the depression went away after a time. I said I would be glad to try to help when he came out of it. Then I played them a recording of one of my laryngectomy patients who had excellent esophageal speech and demonstrated some of my own. I'm not sure that Mr. G. even heard it but his wife left with some hope.

When they returned some two weeks later he was a different man. "Tell me what I have to do!" he wrote. "I'm not programmed to fail." But when I began to outline how we would have to proceed and why, Mr. G. became very impatient and angry. He grabbed the pencil and wrote "Show me!" So I played him the same recording of the excellent esophageal speaker because I knew I could not do it as well. I've learned to do a pretty good job on a few short sentences but my larynx always gets in the way. "No, no," he wrote. "Show me!" And so I gave him some of the best esophageal speech I could burp at that moment. Though he made a face of disgust, he immediately tried to imitate me and, of course, failed completely. His reaction was one of fury. Mr. G. couldn't make a sound but I could see the cursing on his moving lips. He grabbed the pencil again, broke its point by pressing it too hard, threw it on the floor and banged his fist on the table and then against his head, his face livid with rage. I stayed very calm, got him another pencil, and waited for the next written message. "To hell with that! What's this other machine or apparatus that I can talk with? Do you have one?"

Before he was shown the electro-larynx in the desk, I tried to verbalize his feelings of frustration and to help him understand that no laryngectomee could possibly master esophageal speech immediately, that a fairly long training period would be necessary, but that most listeners and most laryngectomees seemed to prefer it. I might as well have saved my breath. I could hear him panting through the stoma hole in his neck and see the gauze pad over it flopping as his irritation grew. "Skip the goddam lecture," he wrote. "Give me the machine." So I took out the electrolarynx, demonstrated how it was used, and placed it carefully against his throat. "Just say 'ah,' then count to three," I requested, as I depressed the buzzer button. It was a mistake. I should have said the same thing first myself so he could know how it would sound. Well, he did say "ah" and counted to five before he grabbed the instrument away from me and flung it against the wall. He was crying— silently of course—as he stormed out of the room. I didn't think he'd come back. But he did return and we did our utmost. Three weeks later, however, he put a bullet through his head. Even now, twenty years later, I keep wondering what else I could have done for Mr. G. The ache of inadequacy has a long life.

the anxious client

Most of the people who come to us for help arrive with some degree of anxiety, and all clinicians must learn how to cope with it. Even when your role is simply that of having to get some essential information from a parent, that first contact has some emotional coloring. Most parents, of course, are a bit nervous, not knowing quite what to expect, but they relax as soon as you reveal yourself as a competent professional and focus the attention on the child's problem. Some beginners start by bombarding the parent with questions immediately, a most unwise procedure.

STUDENT CLINICIAN: May I have your name and age, please?
MOTHER: Mrs. James Brown. I'm thirty-seven.
CLINICIAN: What is your address?
MOTHER: It's 543 Nurrie Road.
CLINICIAN: How old is James Junior?
MOTHER: He'll be six on April 13th.
CLINICIAN: What do you think you did that caused your son's stuttering?
MOTHER: (Long pause) I've tried and tried to think but I just don't know.
CLINICIAN: There's always some reason. Have you ever punished him while he was talking?

This was enough. The supervisor, who had been listening to the interchange, came into the room and took over.

In contrast, an experienced clinician would probably have begun the interview differently—perhaps like this:

CLINICIAN: Mrs. Brown, I'm Miss Carter. I'm sorry you had to wait so long for this appointment. Could I get you a cup of coffee?

MOTHER: No, thank you. I suppose you people are pretty busy.
CLINICIAN: Oh yes. There are a lot of parents like you with children who need our help and it's always good to be able to relieve their concerns. I suppose you're wondering just what sort of information we need and what the other person will be doing when she examines Jimmy. Let me tell you . . .

Most surgeons and dentists know that the fear of the unknown is the first fear that must be dispelled in their patients. They can't and don't tell you everything that might ensue, but they tell you enough about what they will do and about how much it might hurt so that particular fear can be allayed. You may still dread the drill or the knife but these fears are less threatening than the Fear of Fears—the fear of the dark—the fear of the unknown. The speech pathologist must also deal with this fear immediately and in much the same fashion. By providing this procedural information calmly and professionally, he can at the same time reveal that he knows his stuff and is competent.

Parents also come to us with another fear—that they will be blamed for the child's disorder. Many parents are sure that they must have done something, or not done something, that caused the problem. Sometimes they have; sometimes they haven't. In either case, you won't find out till later, if ever, and the wiser procedure is to give immediate absolution anyway. All parents make mistakes. Most of them don't matter—if the child is loved. And so on. By focusing her attention on the child and on the child's problem rather than upon herself, the mother's initial anxiety is relieved. By recognizing that the clinician is not interested in original causes but in the forces that are maintaining the disorder, the parent usually stops worrying about whether he or she's been at fault.

Student clinicians should also recognize the calming effects of "the bedside manner," which a physician once described as the most potent drug in his pharmacopoeia. Some beginners seem to be able to assume this manner from the start; others gain it later. It comes when the beginner stops thinking of her own needs and starts thinking about those of the person she is interviewing. Here are a few adjectives that crudely describe this manner: unhurried, calm, direct, organized, confident, and concerned. Since each of us translate these words into our body language in different ways, there are many "bedside manners" and you will have to discover the one that fits both you and your client.

Now let us turn to therapy and the fears and anxieties of the clients we try to help. Again let me say very emphatically that in many of our clients anxiety is *not* an important part of the clinical problem. All of us have some fears and anxieties, and so do all of our clients, old or young. These anxious feelings come to all of us—from having to live outside Eden. Indeed, a bit of anxiety adds a little pepper to a pot which otherwise might be too bland. As David Harum once opined, "A certain amount of fleas is good for a dog. Keeps him from brooding on being a dog."

But we must also recognize that in this profession all of us will meet many clients whose therapeutic equations contain an important factor of fear, and that often our success or failure will be determined by how we cope with it. Remembering that the tales are of unusual clients, rather than of the ordinary garden variety, let me present them in the hope that you may gain, vicariously, some insightful experience that may prove useful someday.

In my long professional career, I have had to work with many frightened children. Some were the victims of child abuse; some had intense phobias of widely different origins. But the three most frightened of all were the Wild Children of the Swamp.

When my wife and I lived on a farm where our airport now stands, I used to spend a lot of time hunting the swamplands east of the railroad tracks. Pretty wild country then, in the late 1930s. The area, about four square miles, had only one habitation, a little log shack sitting in a small clearing at the end of a two-rut woods road. When looking for a pothole with some ducks in it once I had seen an old Model T Ford truck there and some dirty kids playing around it. Didn't think much about them—just wondered why anyone would want to live in such an isolated dump.

Then one day I had a visit from our sheriff who said he'd picked up three abandoned kids, none of whom could talk, and he couldn't find even a temporary foster home for them because of their lack of speech. He said they acted like little animals. But he'd managed to find their father, "a dumb clunkerhead named Charley Jones" who told him the mother had run away with some hobo. Anyway, would I see them and see if I could teach them to talk? He'd find some place for them to stay for a short time. I was intrigued but insisted on interviewing the father first.

Charley Jones turned out to be a dirty, nondescript, mentally retarded man of about forty who didn't know what had happened to him. "I ain't done nuthin' wrong, boss," he said. "I just dunno. We wuz gittin along OK over there in the swamp, me, my wife and the kids. I haul junk when I kin git it and I always bring bread and other stuff home for them to eat when I can." He would lose his train of thought and his faded blue eyes would wander. Hard to interview, but gradually I pieced out the story. He'd had a job or part-time job clearing the yards of a paper factory long enough to buy himself the fourth-hand truck, but then he was fired and evicted from the house he'd been renting near the mill. Someone had told him of the shack in the swamp and . . . and . . . How long had he lived there? Charley wasn't sure. Had the children been born there? He tried to remember but shook his head. A long time? He guessed maybe. When and why did his wife leave him? She up and took off with the man. What man, Charley? "Oh, that man bummin' down the railroad track." And then Charley became a bit animated for the first time. "You think I done right, boss?" he asked anxiously. "What did you do, Charley?" "Well, I . . . I seen he was hungry and I give him bread. And he got no place for sleep so I say OK come out of rain. And he stay. And stay. And one night he come in bed and want to be in middle of bed and I say no. And he say yes. And I get my axe and he run. And my woman run with him and I don't see her no more. I feed my kids, Boss. I bring home bread for them. I don't do no wrong. Was wrong to say he no could sleep in middle? Why Sheriff come get me, Boss? Why he take kids? They don't do nothing bad. Just play.'' (I fear I don't capture the language, but perhaps I have communicated Charley's bewilderment and dull innocence.)

So I saw the kids. And my secretary put them in the playroom so I could watch them through the mosquito-screened window then used as a one-way mirror. There were three of them: the oldest Ed, a boy of about seven years with wild eyes; the youngest, a bedraggled little girl of perhaps four, Amy; and the middle one, Carl, who looked pretty normal. (Charley had told me their names but he didn't know their ages) I also asked him if they could talk and he replied that they ''used to . . . a little'' . . . and he said they knew their own names.

As I watched through the screen I saw the three children huddled in a corner like kittens in a cold barn, silent and not moving for almost five minutes. Then the oldest one separated from the tangle and tiptoed all around the edge of the room, listening and watching. Then he motioned the other two to come with him to the door which he found was locked. Then he spied a little blue truck which had been placed under the table (with a ball and other toys), made a dive for it, and suddenly the room was full of wild animals, fighting, snarling, making animal noises of every kind, barking, mewing, shrieking. I knocked on the door and they fled again to huddle in the corner, human again but silently frozen with terror. I sat down in a chair and played with the truck and talked to myself about what I was doing, occasionally giving them a slow smile. I held out a piece of candy but none of them would reach for it. It was an eerie first session.

It was soon apparent that the children had to be dealt with individually, which they were, for two years. The two younger ones responded to the training once they had been gentled and shown that the clinician could be trusted but I got nowhere with Ed of the wild eyes. He would not try to talk at all and was finally placed in a home for the severely mentally retarded, where I don't think he really belonged. The little girl got a good foster home (once she got enough speech) but did poorly in school. A slow learner. Carl, the middle child, found very little difficulty in acquiring speech, was adopted into a good home and when I last heard had graduated from high school. How did I teach the two younger ones to talk? Much the same way that we taught our own children, through simplified self-talk and parallel talk and a lot of TLC.

All of us should recognize that when a client is full to the brim with extreme anxiety, this anxiety must be allayed if therapy is to be fruitful. No matter what methods are used, any success will be partial and transitory until we deal with it. We work with the whole person, not just the mouth. This is not to say that we must eliminate anxiety entirely, for often we cannot. Far too often it has its origin in springs hidden deep in the swamps of the person's past, springs that neither we nor the client can know. Yet often we can dam or divert some of the tributary streams and so reduce the flood of anxiety enough to teach the client how to cope with his problems. Sometimes, all we can do is to gain time through palliative measures, knowing that anxiety, like any other emotional state, is never constant. It ebbs and flows. When the fear is at the crest of its wave, we can do little, but in the relative calm of the trough, some progress can be made. So we gain time and wait for a better opportunity. It will come.

And meanwhile we provide an island of safety where that client can wait and not be beset by the terror of being naked and alone. There are some clinicians who mock at supportive therapy. I do not. I have seen its healing powers. In the islands of safety which can be contrived, our clients, overwhelmed by forces they can not control, restore and renew themselves and discover strengths that neither we nor they knew they possessed. Over and over, I have been astounded by the potential for healing and fulfillment that resides in the human spirit—even in the saddest of sacks. But they needed that island of safety and they needed support. Let me tell you about Alberto.

Alberto, according to his father, Giuseppe (Joe), had begun to stutter just after his mother died—when he was six years old—but he was nine or ten at the time I began to work with him. A very severe stutterer, Alberto began almost every phrase or sentence with great laryngeal struggling interrupted by a series of short gasps—severe symptoms to find in such a young child.

Since the father reported that Bert had suddenly become much worse, I arranged to see him every day after school. Joe said that he could bring the boy but could not come after him. I said I'd take him home. The father explained that he ran a little family-type Italian restaurant on a side street downtown and the hours from five to eight were his busiest. I asked Joe whether I should bring Bert back to the restaurant or to his home. The boy broke his silence to say "restaurant" and it must have been five minutes before he got it said. I watched the father while the boy struggled and he almost went crazy. Flung up his hands, tried to guess the word, cursed in Italian, prayed, wept, then grabbed my hand and kissed it saying, "You see. You see. You help Alberto, my boy?" I said I'd try.

The therapy was very difficult at first. Bert was as volatile as his father. Couldn't tolerate the slightest bit of pressure or failure without emoting all over the place, sometimes slapping himself in the face, sometimes weeping inconsolably for long periods. I waited calmly for the upheavals to pass, and then returned to the tasks. Little by little, Bert began to calm down and to gain some relief as he learned that he didn't have to squeeze his "speech doors" shut before trying so say something. I reinforced the fluency he did have. For example, we used a lot of harmonica-talk with both of us speaking through the holes of the instruments, a procedure which provided some masking noise and also counteracted his characteristic blockage of airflow.

Once Bert had come to trust me and had achieved enough "easy speech" to be able to communicate without the old struggling, I began to explore the submerged part of the stuttering iceberg in a roundabout way. What could he remember about his mother—or her death? Surprisingly, he showed little emotion. He had very little to say about his mother except that he remembered her as being very nice, not mean, and she was dead in heaven and didn't have to work so hard any more. I probed some more but there was no real pay-dirt in that area. So I went down to the cafe to talk to Giuseppe (Joe) about the conditions at onset. He was glad to see me, kissed my hand again, brought out two bottles of wine, one "for here" and one "to take home." He said Alberto was talking much better to him but not to his mother. His mother?

We had been lax in taking the case history. Joe had remarried and Bert now had a stepmother. The boy's stuttering had begun not after his real mother's death, but after the stepmother arrived on the scene.

Joe told quite a tale. He'd found out after his first wife died that he couldn't handle the restaurant alone because she had done all the cooking. He couldn't find a good Italian cook so he tried doing it himself and hiring someone to wait table and be the cashier. No good! Bert had helped but he was too small. So after trying in vain to find a new wife who could cook Italian, and who wasn't "spoiled like American women," he went back to Italy, found a young girl, tasted her cooking, married her and brought her to Kalamazoo.

How does the old saying go: the best laid eggs of mice and hens aren't always what they're cracked up to be? Or something similar. Anyway, Giuseppe had not chosen wisely. The new wife was a shrew, a hellion, an easy spender, a castrator. Hell to live with but she wasn't lazy and she was a good cook—so the restaurant had flourished. But she was very mean to Bert and his younger brother. Whipped them too much, Joe said. Hated them.

At the end of our next session Bert finally talked about his stepmother. What a torrent of emotion! What a tale! Often he became completely incoherent as one severe stuttering block after another returned to his speech. He told of the many beatings she had given him. He took off his shirt to show me the red-purple welts of the last one (administered with sticks and even a skillet). She had found a piece of string on the carpet when she returned from the cafe the previous night! Bert and his brother always had to come straight home from school and never leave the house even to play in the yard. They had to have the house spotless when she returned. They could not speak except to answer one of her questions while she was in the house—not even to each other. If Bert stuttered he got a hard slap across the mouth. And once when he failed to clean up his plate he had to eat from the garbage can for a week. And once she had punished him for something he couldn't remember—nothing big—by taking him down to the basement, tying him to a post and sticking needles in him. And much more. I asked Bert if his father knew how the stepmother treated him. "Only a little."

I went to the cafe to see Joe. Read him the riot act. Told him if he couldn't make his wife stop abusing the boy, I'd go see the judge and have Bert put in a foster home or something. And that they could put him or his wife in jail too. Scared him good.

Two days later the father came to see me, gesturing wildly and very upset. "What I can do, Doc? What I can do?" He told me that he had given his wife a good beating the night after our conference to "teach her how to act" but then that night he had awakened from a deep sleep to find her standing over him with a knife. He beat her up again but Joe was a frightened man. "What I can do, Doc?" Playing God, I told him to get a new cook and a divorce.

He did. His wife fought the action, however, and I had to go to court to give hearsay testimony to the judge in his chambers that I could not provide during the formal hearing. The judge, a good man, believed me but suggested that Bert testify for himself, a decision I opposed because of the stress on the boy's speech. Somehow the problem was resolved. Evidently the wife's attorney interviewed Bert and saw immediately that his case was lost. Anyway, Joe was granted custody, and the woman went off to live with relatives in Detroit. In only a few weeks, Bert's speech was almost free from stuttering. Just a few miniature laryngeal blockings and those only under strong communicative pressure. I rechecked him at intervals sporadically for over a year and found no recurrence of the former stuttering behaviors.

But a few years later, Bert came to my office to tell me that his father was going to remarry the woman. How did he know? Was he sure? Yes. I tore down to the restaurant to confront Giuseppe. Yes, he was going to marry her again. She had learned her lesson. And he had to have someone who could cook Italian.

"Oh, oh!" I thought. "Here we go again. Bert will be sure to relapse." But Bert didn't. The time and the island of safety and our support had enabled him to grow strong enough to cope.

Thirty years later Bert is a successful business man. Occasionally he stutters mildly. No hard struggling. No gasps. Just hesitates.

We are far more than trainers of tongues.

Anxiety and fear, though closely related, are not the same, the difference lying in the focus or lack of it. When the mother bear chases you away from her cubs, it is fear you feel; when you must wander the deep woods at night, it is anxiety that sends the shivers up your back. Psychiatrists speak of anxiety as being free-floating, as generalized apprehension, and describe fear as being specific. Both have in common the expectation of approaching unpleasantness. Both can vary widely in intensity—all the way from mild uneasiness to utter panic. A person in the throes of a severe anxiety attack is not a pleasant sight. The breathing is disturbed, with hyperventilation, or shuddering inhalations and gasps. The face is pale, yet perspiration may cover it. The eyes are as wide as those of a frightened horse. The heart beats erratically. Yet the clinician must stay steady and strong until the attack passes, for the relationship thereafter will be much closer. Once the client knows that you have not abandoned him when he most needed you, you will find you can be much more effective.

Though these experiences are fortunately rather rare, you are certain to have to cope with the fears of some of your clients if you hope to help them. We have known lispers who dreaded every approaching /s/ words. We have worked with children with clefts of the lip and palate who preferred to play stupid in school and play alone on the playground because of their fear of peer mockery and rejection. Adults often have told us of their fear of exposing their speech deviancies. "It's those damned eyeballs," one of them said. "The moment I start to say something they pop out all over the place—and then they look away. I live in a world full of eyeballs." Another said, "It's that sudden dead silence I dread. Everybody's talking along, and then someone asks me a casual question and I answer. Suddenly all the talk stops and there I am, naked in my abnormality." A woman with spastic dysphonia wept. "I start out all right for a few words and then my voice fails. And then I see my listener first surprised, then concerned, then pitying me. The pity is the worst. It demeans me. I fear that look of pity more than anything. I'm now getting so I fear even trying to talk."

But the clients with the most fears will be your confirmed stutterers. They show fears of speaking situations, fears of certain words, fears of certain sounds, fears of relapse—yes, even fear of having fear, for they believe that the more they fear, the more they stutter. Many of these stutterers live in almost constant fear and yet they cannot adapt to it because they have periods of fluency, too. As one of them said, "I wish I were blind, or crippled, or deaf because then I could get used to it. But I live under the dangling sword, knowing that it will fall and cut me, but never really being sure just when." These stutterers devise intricate strategies for avoiding these feared sounds, words, and situations. They intently scan their listeners, their own sounds and words for danger signs. The world of the stutterer is a strange one, but you must be able to enter it through the door of understanding.

The stutterer's fears can also be very intense. We have felt their pulse rates increase from 78 to 130 as they entered a classroom to speak before a group. We have seen a college student fight for the courage to pick up the telephone, and then, when someone answered, fling it to the floor and crouch sobbingly in a corner of the room. In many ways these stuttering fears are self-fulfilling prophecies. As the stutterer approaches a feared speaking situation, he rehearses what he is going to say, tasting almost each word for probability of stuttering, selecting substitutions of easy words for hard ones, rearranging them, avoiding them by circumlocutions, inserting carrier words or phrases, making contingency plans for fears that might flare up at the last moment, hunting for possible distractions or ways of disguising any stuttering that might occur, and constantly calculating the probabilities of distress. If this seems unbelievable to you, to a severe stutterer it is the way he lives each day. Caught in the meshes of this net of fear, the stutterer struggles to escape and avoid, only to find that he is entangled further. The more he avoids, the more he fears, and the more he stutters!

Many stutterers flee; some fight. A few just quit the verbal world altogether. One of my friends, a brilliant, lovely man, walked into the Iowa River after being interviewed for a job (and rejected), then came out, put on his shoes and walked back in again. We saw his footprints before we found the body. And I knew a stutterer who became a Trappist monk and swore an oath of eternal silence. Somewhere in the Ozark Mountains there is a hermit who does not talk to anyone. He was once a client of mine, one that I fought hard to heal, but lost. I don't blame him at all and I don't blame myself. I did my damndest with what I had. It wasn't enough. Better to be a hermit than to go through life stuttering like he did. Each must find a lifestyle that fits. So let me tell you about Raoul of the Bayou de la Fange.

I was in Louisiana one March, conducting a week-long workshop in stuttering for the speech pathologists in the area. My lectures, demonstration therapy, and discussion sessions took most of the mornings, but my afternoons and evenings were free and it was a lovely land. (All of us should have at least two springs each year, and there was still snow in Michigan.) The group was fairly large, perhaps a hundred or so, and the participants were eager to learn. Most of them were young, attractive clinicians but I especially noticed one person, a white-haired lady who always sat in the back row and hung on every dubious word I uttered, furiously taking notes. She kept to herself and did not fraternize with the other clinicians during coffee break, nor did she take any part in the discussions. At the end of the Thursday session, however, she came up and introduced herself.

She was not a speech therapist, she said. She had come to hear me in the hope that she could help her forty-year-old son who stuttered and who had isolated himself on their plantation since quitting high school at sixteen. She told me that Raoul talked as little as possible to anyone, spent his days in his room listening to the radio, or reading or wandering the fields and swamp. Perhaps if he saw me and heard me, another person who had stuttered, speaking so fluently, Raoul might have some hope, might break out of his isolation. She hesitated to ask, but could I, would I come to their home to see Raoul? She warned me that he might not come downstairs, might refuse to speak to me, but would I please come? Of course I agreed.

Her chauffeur picked me up at two o'clock that afternoon and drove me thirty miles to a landing on the Bayou de la Fange where we took a launch to the plantation. The driver explained that it was easier that way because of the muddy roads at that time of year and that Mme. F. thought I would enjoy the boat ride. I certainly did. The trees hung heavily with moss, there were strange shrubs in full bloom in the sunny places, and an incredible variety of birds sang everywhere.

The house was very old and very beautiful. Mme. F. welcomed me graciously and showed me a huge book of historic homes in which the house was pictured. The book said that it had been built in the days of the Napoleons and that the roof tiles had come from France by sailing ship. Both she and her husband were of French descent, very proud to be Creoles. He was a consulting engineer, specializing in the erection and management of sugar refineries and soon to retire. He would be joining us shortly. She led me through the huge drawing room filled with antique furniture into a little alcove overlooking the garden and then excused herself. "I must persuade Raoul to join us—if I can." I suggested that perhaps she should leave us alone after he came so we could speak more freely of our common problem.

More than twenty minutes elapsed before Raoul entered the alcove and sat down. A large man, almost fat, he wouldn't shake hands as we were introduced. So I did all the talking at first, revealing myself, telling of my own experiences as a severe stutterer, verbalizing the feelings of the stutterers I had known and helped. I showed Raoul how I used to stutter and demonstrated how fluent I had become. I verbalized the joys of being freed from a tongue that had been so badly twisted. No hard sell at all, just a calm, almost casual, presentation of factual material so that Raoul would know that I understood what it was like to be a stutterer.

Throughout this long soliloquy—and that is what it was, for the man didn't say a word—I was watching his body language closely. At first it appeared to reflect complete indifference and detachment; then some flickers of attention appeared, then some alarm, and finally some real interest in the subject. When these latter signals occurred I told him I wasn't there to try to get him to undertake any therapy, that I had come only because of his mother's concern and because he probably needed some hope. It was only then that he began to talk.

"I know," Raoul said, "my mother is worrying about what will happen to me when she and my father die and I am left here alone. They are getting old, yes." Raoul didn't stutter very frequently nor at all severely as he said this. He told me *he* wasn't worried. He lived only one day at a time. He was never bored. His main hobby was baseball. Although he had never seen a professional team, Raoul knew the batting averages and earned run averages of all the players on several teams and followed them closely on the radio and in the newspapers. He made predictions, bets with himself, on the outcome of the games. It was almost an obsession but it passed the time away. When there was no baseball, there was hunting and fishing and reading. Why talk and suffer? Here he was happy, safe. The world "out there" was full of evil and danger. He wanted no part of it. Here on the plantation he didn't have to talk if he didn't want to; "out there" he would be as miserable as he'd been in high school. To hell with it. He shook hands with me, smiled, and left. I lit my pipe and wiped my brow.

When his mother came in, she took one look at my face and knew. "Ah, mon fils," she said, patting my arm, "it was the long chance. I know you tried. Raoul, he has lived this way too long. Now you must meet my husband and share our pleasantness." A maid came in with a tray of sweets and tiny egg-shell thin cups. "These are from old France," she said, "and now you must know the coffee of that time." The maid put a tiny bit of the very black coffee in each fragile cup, then a teaspoon of boiling water over it, then a bit more coffee, then another teaspoon of water and so on until the little cup was full. Then brown raw sugar and thick cream. The best coffee I have ever tasted or will taste in my whole life. Raoul's father, a gay spirit, joined us and had some too. No further mention of the son—just gaiety and civilité. The father told tales of the Creoles; I told about the French Canadians of the forest village where I spent my boyhood. We even knew and sang the same old song of the voyageurs:

> "Oh ze wind she blo from ze nort',
> And ze wind, she blo some more,
> But you won't get drown on Lac Champlain
> So long you stay on ze shore."

I don't know what happened to Raoul when his parents died and he had to leave that shore of his.

Other clients find other ways beside avoidance and escape for easing the tyranny of the speech anxiety that pervades their lives. Some of them turn to booze; some to compulsive and indiscriminate sex, some to drugs, and so they compound their difficulties. Some find relief in feeding and become so grossly fat that additional rejection is experienced. A few become hypochondriacs, transferring some of the worry from their speech to their health. One of our clients with dysphonia was a sleeper, spending as many as twenty hours dozing in her bed, yet constantly suffering from a fatigue that no medication could ameliorate. Lee Travis, one of the pioneers in our field, once said that "a speech therapist had to know everything about everything" to serve his clients. There have been times when the need to be informed about all of these accessory problems has been burdensome, but again: *unto their needs!* The tragedy of these wasted, twisted lives is that most of them could have been prevented had these people received the professional help they needed early enough. Sometimes I think that if I could begin again I would work only with children. But then again, we must remember that most of our adult clients have not had these problems except in miniature and that once they were helped to learn to speak fairly normally, they led good lives.

the guilt-ridden client

In the course of a long career I have interviewed many hundreds of parents of children with severe speech disorders. Perhaps there were a few of them who came without any feeling of guilt, but I cannot remember who they were. Most of their reactions could be placed on the lower end of the continuum of embarrassment-shame-guilt, but these parents all seemed to feel responsible in some way for the fact that their child did not speak normally. Having been a parent myself, I have a keen awareness that we are bound to make mistakes in the way we interact with our children. There are always sins of commission or omission but most of them play no part in the causation or maintenance of the child's speech difficulties. Parents, however, do not know this. They blame themselves, and they blame each other, and our society tends, unfortunately, to make them feel that this blame is justified. Among the Eskimo and the Polynesian cultures, a speech disorder or any other kind of disability is viewed in the same manner as a lopsided nose—as an act of God. Too bad, but they were just born that way, and no parent feels guiltily responsible. Not so in our culture.

Accordingly, when you must interview a parent of a child with a speech disorder, you should keep these parental guilt feelings in mind. You should define your own role as a *problem* solver and investigator, rather than as that of a judge or priest. Show that you understand their feelings but that you will not blame them for anything they have done or not done. When they find that you are also willing to accept some of the responsibility for the child's problem, they will find great relief. And then they will tell you more, sometimes much more than they had intended to reveal, sometimes more than they should have disclosed. (Some Pandora's boxes should not be opened.) When the parent or client is spilling more traumatic information than he is ready or really willing to disclose and which he will later regret, he will watch us closely for any sign of rejection.

Sometimes he may invite us to join him in his self-blaming, and these moments provide a good opportunity for defining our professional role as an objective, permissive, and accepting consultant. We will not judge. We will simply try to understand so that we can help solve the problem.*

When both parents come to the diagnostic interview, it is preferable to interview them separately, then see them both together for a summary and recommendations. These joint sessions have often resulted in some beautiful family fights, each parent accusing the other, with frequent displays of strong emotion. Inevitably the father or the mother will try to get you to take sides, and the only safe course is to show that you desire to understand both but only so that you can help the child. Though occasionally the problem lies in the parents rather than in the child, the latter must be your focus. "Problem, problem. Who's got the problem?" The answer is usually that all of them have, but no one ever really can be sure.

Now let us turn to the clients themselves and the role that guilt and shame can play in their difficulties and treatment. First of all, hostility, anxiety, and guilt are not independent entities. They all involve unpleasant emotional arousal and can be categorized under the heading of negative emotion. The physiologists tell us that they have found few differences in the glandular secretions of these different emotional states, and certainly we find hostility, fear and guilt blended together in different proportions clinically. The stutterer may fear the feelings of shame, anxiety, and anger, and experience all of them at the same time. A hostile client with vocal nodules may feel guilty for smearing you with that hostility, and simultaneously he may fear that you will dismiss him from therapy.

Moreover, just as anxiety can convert itself into hostility when it becomes too unbearable, so either of these emotional states can change into guilt. And then there can come a desire for penance and punishment. Let me tell you of a very anxious little girl who found some easing of her anxiety by being bad. We shall call her Eva.

The influence of negative emotion as a precipitant of stuttering has always interested me. Usually that emotional state is fear or anxiety, but it can also be anger, guilt or any other of the psychological acids. Eva, a pretty little girl, aged eight, was brought to me by her aunt with whom she was staying in our city that summer. The aunt, a warm, loving person, insisted that Eva had not stuttered once when talking with her although the girl had stuttered badly at home in Chicago and also when talking to her mother during the latter's two

---

*Although I usually take a few notes during my interviews with parents and clients, I have found that it is unwise to do so when "hot material" is being divulged. Don't change the subject suddenly, or become transfixed, when the father says of his stuttering son, "I caught the dirty little bastard behind the barn masturbating." Instead suggest, "I suppose Jim has done some other things you didn't like, too." And keep looking at the parent as he replies.

visits to Kalamazoo. When we examined Eva, we found no sign of the stuttering. Indeed, she was one of the most fluent children of her age we have ever known.

With some difficulty, because Eva's parents ran a little family grocery store in the Chicago slums, we managed to interview them at length one Sunday afternoon and to corroborate the aunt's testimony. In the same conversational setting Eva would be completely fluent when addressing us, or the aunt, yet stutter wretchedly when speaking to her father and especially to her mother, showing long, gagging, almost vomiting behaviors, mainly on the first words of her utterances to them. There seemed to be a curious lack of affect or emotion when she stuttered. Eva could have a very long retching struggle and it didn't seem to bother her at all. There was no avoidance and she maintained perfect eye contact with her parents throughout her severe blockings. In contrast, they were visibly upset, the mother reacting with evident irritation. We told the aunt to take Eva for an ice cream cone and to return in an hour while we interviewed the parents.

It was a long, troublesome interview with many false trails that led to nothing meaningful, but eventually the picture clarified. The "stuttering" had begun just after an illness (scarlet fever) when Eva was six years old, one that required a long convalescence. "Well, that was not quite true," the father softly said. "Eva had occasionally shown some hesitation even before she got the scarlet fever." "No, she hadn't," said the mother angrily. After all, *she* was the one who had to take care of the kid and she knew! When I reflected some of the hostility in her voice by saying something about the burdens of parenthood, a torrent of abusive reproach directed at her husband ensued. She gave him purple hell and at length. He hunched his shoulders, rolled his eyes back in a gesture that seemed to say "Thar she blows again!" and waited for the roily river to make its way to sea.

Since I have found that such outbursts often provide more useful information than the most skillful questioning can reveal, I egged her on a bit. Anyway here is the picture that finally outlined itself. The mother was pregnant when they married. She had been raised in comfortable family circumstances but her family had rejected her totally when she became pregnant and all she had known since then had been struggle and poverty. In her view, the grocery store was her one hope of making enough money to get out of the slums, and she had worked day and night to manage it (and her husband) so that she could do so. Then, at just about the time when she could see enough success to hope that they could sell out and move, Eva got sick, almost died, and the mother had to stay home to take care of her. While she was doing so, her husband made a mess of the business, got far back in debt again, didn't take care of the customers, etc., etc. He was not only financially irresponsible but just plain stupid, among many other things. It was she who had the brains and the energy; he was nothing but a burden. Although I felt sorry for her husband, I let her flow, holding constantly in my head the essential question: "But what does this have to tell me about the reason for Eva's situation-bound stuttering?"

Gradually it became very apparent that the mother felt as much hostility for the girl as she did for her husband. If Eva hadn't come along, and damn him for seducing her, she would be having the old comforts, clothes, friends and activities of her former life; she wouldn't have to slave and grub down there in the slums trying desperately to find a way out. "When I hear Eva stutter, I could puke," she told me. Though I remembered how the girl retched when she stuttered, I was sympathetic. "And then just about the time you felt the business was beginning to make money and you could escape. . . ." The mother didn't wait for me to finish the statement. She poured out her hate until the office was flooded with it. Finally the man couldn't take another bit. "Shut your goddam mouth, you bitch!", he yelled. "I love that kid and I won't have you saying things like that."

She turned on him in such fury that once again he slumped in his chair. "So she's sweet, is she? She just knows how to work you. Sweet, hey? How about that time when you took the money out of our savings account and bought that new car and had it all shined and polished and she dug up the rotten meat you'd put under that one scraggly rose bush for fertilizer and smeared it all over your new car. And smeared it all over her hair too. Sweet, you say? Sweet? You spoil her rotten. Always. Lovey dovey, you two. Even when she did that, who had to spank her good? Not him." That's how the encounter went for nearly two hours.

Rarely is there a perfect solution to a problem, but there is always something that can be done. Somehow the child had to be removed temporarily from the parents, especially the mother, while we tried to reinforce the fluency she already had, and to help her build barriers against rejection. Fortunately, Eva's aunt was childless so she agreed to keep her for at least the six months that appeared to be needed. I instituted a program of play therapy so that the girl could act out some of her conflicts. She was desensitized to hierarchies of many rejections, using an older female student as a mother substitute while I played the father's role myself. (We finally got a recurrence of some of Eva's old stuttering occasionally when going up the steps of the hierarchy too fast but it was easily extinguished and it was repetitive, not gagged.) Meanwhile, the mother, freed from her hated albatross, worked like a fiend in the store and made it a growing success again. The six months grew to a year, and then another. Eva made the transition to a new school easily. No stuttering there, nor in her new home either. I tapered off our sessions and finally terminated the case, leaving the final disposition to the aunt as to whether or not Eva would ever go back to Chicago.

But I'll never forget one of our play sessions. It was based on our mutual verbalizing of the thoughts of father, mother and baby dolls as we played with them. The parent dolls fought and argued a lot, Eva always preferring to hold the mother and always winning the arguments. (She used an angry, nasty voice.) Often she would tell me when I was holding the father doll to spank the baby hard because she had done one bad thing or another. When she tired of the play, I finally asked her what her real mother was like and if she had ever spanked her. "No," said Eva, vehemently. "No, no!" The girl then proceeded to paint a picture of her mother as the nicest, most loving, beautiful woman in the whole world. Her father was OK but her mother (that evil, nasty shrew who had hated the girl for years) was perfect beyond perfection. Eva was serenely sure of this.

It was easy to understand that, holding to this illusion, the girl gained a precarious security. All of us need to idealize the ones on whom we depend. Were she to admit the obvious fact that her mother was an unpleasant, vicious old devil who hated her, Eva would know she was in jeopardy. But how could she maintain such an illusion in the light of the mother's constant punishment and rejection? By justifying the mother's behavior—by being bad, by smearing the new car, by doing things that made the mother's punishing behavior quite reasonable. Was Eva's revolting kind of stuttering one more way of saying that it was she who was bad, not her mother?

You decide. But before you do, let me tell you one more thing that happened in our play therapy. I had not heard a bit of her stuttering for months, even when I inserted bits of rejection into our interaction. Then one day, when I held the mother doll while Eva held the baby doll, I made the "mother" spank the baby hard and portray a lot of angry rejection. Eva made the baby doll cry terribly and say "No, no Mummy. Please don't hit me, Mummy." And she stuttered gaggingly in her old way on almost every word.

In our culture, alas, speech disability or physical disability tends to evoke negative reactions from those who are not disabled. Children on the playground can be very cruel to those whose differences are visible or audible. Deviancy is penalized unless the person has other assets that can override or compensate for the handicap. The mockery, the labeling through name calling, the overt or covert rejections comprise the gauntlet that most deviants must run.

I remember still my own pain when strangers came to our dining table and I had to eat in the kitchen so that my stuttering would not embarrass my parents. And I recall vividly the look on my father's face after a hard bout of stuttering, a look of utter disgust and despair. And I also remember well what he said, not once but several times: "My God, I'll have to support you all my life." The tragedy of such statements and reactions is that the child becomes suffused with a guilt that may shape his entire life. Even one cruel remark may reverberate for years with such devastating effects on self-esteem that any therapy will be ineffective.

"I have never had a right hand," said a cerebral palsied girl named Sue. "I lost it in grade school when one morning I reached for a piece of toast at the breakfast table and my sister said in revulsion, 'Take that claw off the plate. I can't bear to look at it.' Jerrie never said anything like that again, but I've never been able to forget. I don't have a right hand; I have a claw!" How to respond? I took that claw, kissed it and turned it into a hand again. But this occurred far along in therapy so let me go back to the beginning of the story.

Sue came to me when she was a senior in high school. She had the variety of cerebral palsy termed tension athetosis and her handicap was a very severe one. Sue's speech, when I first examined her, was almost unintelligible. The voice was strained and trembling. Her articulation was very distorted. When Sue was asked to write something on a pad, she could hardly pick up the pencil and when she finally managed to do so, using both hands, it jerked all over the paper in utter sprawl. Her gait was awkward and unstable. But it was her facial expression that really got me after I had learned to disregard the shaky writhing of her mouth. It seemed to be utterly sad, resigned and hopeless. It is hard to see that look on a client's face (perhaps because I wore it too long myself), so I said I'd do all I could to help her. Even as I said it, I wondered whether I had any right to sign the invisible contract, and if I were doing it for her or for my own needs. Yet there was something about Sue that was difficult to put into words, but which spoke silently of hidden strength and courage. Despite all her tremors and jerks, she kept trying until she did what she had to do. She did the best she could.

Then there was also the fact that Sue had somehow been able to go almost all the way through high school, a feat that seemed impossible considering her handicap. I interviewed her teachers, and then her mother, a big-busted, formidable woman. The teachers all said that Sue could not recite at all but that she was very intelligent and fulfilled every assignment by typing it (and also her test answers) alone in a room by herself. She always needed more time than the average student, they said, but they had given it to her. But how could she type with such a disability in coordination? One of the teachers gave me the key. "Sue just can't function when she is on display," she said. "When she is alone by herself she can do almost anything. Though it takes her a long time, she always gets it done." The mother corroborated this information and added that when Sue talked to herself or to her pets she talked much better. Not normally, but much better.

I didn't know much about cerebral palsy or "Little's Disease," as it was then called, so I read everything I could find about it—which was little indeed. I admitted my ignorance to physician friends and asked their counsel. Most of them had little to offer. Their general advice was to teach the girl to relax but they had little hope that it could be done. No wonder it was called "Little's Disease." Thus unprepared, I began.

The first thing I discovered was that Sue's expression had been misread completely. She was not resigned, hopeless or helpless at all; instead she was terribly ashamed of being the way she was. Actually, as her success in school despite all odds had demonstrated, Sue was very strong-willed—like her mother, she said. She didn't know how she would be able to do it, but somehow she would find some way to be self-supporting and to have a good life. She knew that to achieve this goal she would need as much education as she could get. I found a very strong person inside that very tense, contorted exterior.

We began with relaxation training, following models found in the few books, mostly from England and Germany, that I possessed. These were based mainly upon strong verbal suggestions given to the patient lying on a cot. It was miserable, time-consuming work, replete with failure after failure, but every so often Sue would really calm down, the flailing would cease, her face would stop contorting, and then for a short period, if she spoke very softly, her speech became almost normal. This gave us great hope but it soon became evident that the problem was not going to be solved in this way. While Sue could relax when with me in the therapy room, any attempt to maintain the state in outside situations failed completely. I tried all sorts of hierarchies (we called them graded-situations then) to effect some transfer but without the slightest success. Whenever Sue had to talk to someone else she became so hypertense it was hard to believe she had had any therapy at all. I was discouraged; Sue was not. She said I had shown her that she could talk well to at least one person. Somehow we would find a way.

By this time we had achieved a satisfying clinical relationship. Sue trusted me, and for my part, I was completely open and honest with her. I told her very little was known about cerebral palsy but I would try to learn more and share with her every crumb of information obtainable. I asked her to teach me to identify and assume her postures, her foci of tension, her spasmodic movements. One winter morning when I was attempting to imitate her difficulties while walking on ice and snow, we both realized at the same instant that she fell so often because, when she began to slip, she *lifted* her right foot rather than putting it down. So we practiced falling differently, unaware that a big football player was watching us until he charged in furiously and threatened to knock my head off for tripping "that poor cripple." Sue told him off and her speech was fluent and well-articulated. We sat down on a snowbank and looked at each other in amazement. When I asked her why she had been able to talk so well at that moment, Sue said it was because for once she wasn't thinking about herself as a shameful thing.

Well, that remark changed the course of therapy. We began to explore her feelings and history at the same time that she was trying to control and lessen her bodily tension, first on the cot, then in a chair, and finally as we talked and walked. Rather simplistically, we set up as a hypothesis the proposition that shame and guilt were the sources of the tension that comprised the major portion of her physical and speech handicaps. "All right," said Sue. "I shall conquer that shame. What do I do first?" "I'm a helluva priest," I answered, "but I think it's time for confession. Let's dig up all the dead cats and lay them on the table. What experiences created these constant feelings of shame and guilt?"

I cannot possibly recount them all. There was the tale of the claw and a hundred other of the same ilk. Sue's mother had always hated her and been ashamed of her. The father had deserted the family when she was four years old, and the mother had to go back to teaching, a profession she hated, in order to support Sue and her older sister. "I've always been the burden," Sue wept. "Every piece of bread I ate made me feel guilty. Every time my mother brushed my hair—she always brushed it hard and viciously—I could feel the hate. She always took my sister to the store—but not me." She told me of many humiliations inflicted by her older sister. She recounted the looks of revulsion and disgust she had seen on her mother's face. Sue told of the time that she had learned by herself to ride a tricycle owned by a neighboring child and had been yanked off the sidewalk by her mother who had yelled at her, "Don't make a spectacle of yourself, you horrible child." Over and over again I heard the refrain: "I've got to get away. I've got to support myself."

So I persuaded The Madam, my wife, who was then pregnant with our first child, to let Sue live with us for a time. Over the years, we have taken in fourteen of these lost and desperate souls for many months at a time, and they have greatly enriched our lives, though at some cost to us in stress as they acted out their own family conflicts. Sue's mother was very glad to see her go.

Sue enrolled half time in college but the rest of the time she participated in all our family activities. We took her with us everywhere. We insisted that she drink from our finest china cups and do the dishes afterwards, and to the devil with the breakage. She learned to ice skate on our pond. And we bathed her in humor, appreciation, and affection. No pity. No rejection. No guilt. Just do the best you can. In this environment Sue flowered beyond belief and although the athetosis remained almost intact, the tension subsided, and with it went most of the jerks and contortions. Her speech improved rapidly enough to allow her to recite in class as well as to converse with her fellow students. She even had a date or two, received a good scholarship so she could finish college and made plans so she could live in the dormitory after she left us.

Sue graduated in special education and taught in schools for crippled children until she retired. A wonderful teacher, everyone said, and a wonderful person. She was asked, many years after she left our home, if she could pinpoint any one experience that had been crucial. At first she said no, that it was having someone who had faith in her and who had helped her stop feeling like a burden and a monster. But then she added this: "Yes, I think there was one after all. It was when you and Mrs. Van came back from the hospital and you put that tiny baby in my spastic arms."

Guilt and punishment are closely intertwined. Each will breed the other.* If the punishment is not forthcoming from society, then the guilty person will contrive some way of punishing himself. Confession, penance, absolution is the usual therapeutic sequence. This is why some of our clients have used their abnormal speech behaviors as punishment, as flagellation, hoping thereby to find some relief from their intense feelings of guilt. Clinicians should know that in these cases, if the guilt is not dealt with and ameliorated, the removal of the abnormal speech can create other self-punishing behaviors. These clients are not commonly found but here is one.

Phil, an undergraduate student in our university, was majoring in special education. His basic problem involved phonation, with falsetto, pitch breaks, and intermittent aphonia being the major characteristics. Phil had not referred himself to our clinic. Indeed, he came to us very reluctantly and only because his academic counselor told him bluntly that he would either have to improve his voice or leave the curriculum, that he was completely unemployable as any kind of teacher.

An odd voice and an odd man! When Phil first came in, he was completely aphonic and insisted on writing all his communication. When I told him that even when persons lost their voices they could always whisper, he immediately showed that he could do so too. A bit later, after I heard him clear his throat and produce a brief bit of normal phonation, I told him authoritatively that I would massage his larynx, loosen the tension, and that he could then say "ah." This he did immediately and was able to speak other sentences aloud very easily but in a mono-pitched high falsetto.

Using some more hocus pocus and suggestion, I next sought to lower the pitch and to get the normal phonation which had been heard when he had cleared his throat. This was only occasionally successful. The good voice lasted for only two or three words, then ended in a sudden pitch break upwards into the falsetto again. At the end of our first session Phil was asked to write a detailed autobiography and to include as much material about the nature and onset of his voice problem as he could remember. Apathetically, he agreed to do so. When Phil left, I wondered if I would see him again and I tried to organize my first impressions. The dominant one was the lack of affect. No emotion. Passivity. Little energy in posture, movements or voice. Listless. A psychogenic dysphonia? As always, I cautioned myself to wait until more information became available before making that diagnosis.

---

*This is why we must be very careful in using punishment in behavior modification programs.

Although our next appointment was several days away, I was surprised when my secretary handed me a large thick envelope from Phil the following morning. It was his autobiography, thirty pages long, and an accompanying note said that he had stayed up all night writing it. A most curious document. The first twenty-nine pages covered his early life in minute detail. It was full of trivial information about his childhood pets, chores, school teachers, Boy Scout and church activities, and vacations with his parents. He even devoted a page to describing a valentine he had sent to his mother. He was an only child. He had been raised in a happy home. And so on. Then on the thirtieth and last page he said only that his parents had died when he was in high school, that an uncle and aunt had adopted him and it was about this time that the voice problem had begun. That was all.

Many sessions ostensibly devoted to voice therapy occurred before Phil came to trust me enough to tell the rest of the tale. An incoherent storm of utterance, half-whispered, half full of falsetto and pitch breaks, sometimes only pantomimed, it was difficult to understand. Something about his getting up one cold night and putting gasoline instead of fuel oil into the heater of the little cottage where the family lived and the terrible explosion and the parents trapped in the upper bedroom, and how in the terror of escape he had not thought to get the ladder and . . . and . . . and they died. He could hear their screams yet.

Phil told me he had run across the field to the neighbors but couldn't speak, just make motions, and they couldn't understand. Would have been too late anyway. For months he couldn't talk at all. Or sleep or eat, so he said. I was the first person he had told what had really happened. His aunt had taken him to a child guidance clinic where he had seen a psychiatrist whom he didn't like or trust and in whom he could not confide. He had told a preacher part of the story but had lost his nerve and could not tell the rest. I was the first to know what had really happened . . . that he had killed his parents in their sleep, that he had burned them to death. I had to read Phil's lips to understand that last utterance.

How should one respond at such a moment? I have heard many confessions, though few as traumatic as Phil's, and I still do not know how I *should* respond. All I know is what one does at the moment—stay with the poor devil; be steady; try hard as hell to understand as deeply as I can what the experience must have meant to him. No judging whatsoever. Sharing. Showing that I feel honored that he could see fit to confide in me. Showing that he no longer need bear his burden alone.

But was this not a case for a psychiatrist rather than a speech pathologist? The history of muteness following the tragedy and the intermittent aphonia under communicative stress were pretty good evidence of hysterical dysphonia. The falsetto and its accompanying pitch breaks might possibly be viewed as due to the need to remain the happy child and youth he had been before the trauma. Both pointed to referral. Yet in my experience I had often known vocal and other deviancies to persist long after the original cause had lost its effect. Voices can become habitual too. Nevertheless, the decision was made to refer him to a psychiatrist. Phil had no money to afford private psychotherapy so he was sent to our university psychiatrist, who promptly sent him back to me. "Hysterical aphonia—prognosis poor. My function is crisis intervention. I don't have time to work with him. Suggest you refer him to Dr. So-and-so." But we had referred other clients to Dr. So-and-so and had been more impressed with his rapacity than his competence, so that avenue was closed. Although I had been psychoanalyzed myself and, as a clinical psychologist, had both training and experience in psychological counseling, I was reluctant to take Phil on as a patient. My profession was speech pathology.

When in our next conference I tried to tell him I could not accept him as a client and why, Phil suddenly began to cry and I heard the constrained but deep-toned sobbing of a strong, not a weak, man. Then he became mute, but over and over again he repeated something in pantomime that I could not understand. Finally, when he was offered a pencil and paper, he wrote what he had been trying to say: "Help me! Help me if you can!"

So we began. A detailed account of our work together cannot be presented here but it was a combination of voice therapy and psychotherapy, the emphasis on each varying from session to session. At first nothing was done about the falsetto or pitch breaks, but we concentrated instead on helping Phil produce low-pitched phonation at will mainly because the muteness seemed to be the feature of his problem causing the most distress. And, of course, it was probably very symbolic of the conflict that had not been resolved. I made sure that Phil had more than one way of voluntarily being able to achieve voice, so that if one procedure failed or lost its effectiveness he could resort to another. Altogether he found three ways he could do this: by using the vocal fry and smoothing it out into low pitched vocalization, by clearing his throat and humming, and by swallowing to release the tension, then sighing. Hierarchies were set up and practiced repeatedly. First he would just produce a hum or a vowel, then a single word, then a phrase, then a sentence. If a pitch break upward into the falsetto occurred, Phil had to start up the sequence again. A lot of suggestion was used throughout.

But the unique part of the treatment was the use of emotionally loaded material in Phil's vocal exercises. Each night he had to write out for me the answers to certain questions dealing with the fire in which his parents had died or with Phil's feelings of guilt: "How did the gasoline get in the fuel oil can?" "Describe the explosion." "Try to put into words your first feelings after the accident occurred." Then, from his accounts, I would select a key word, phrase or sentence as the vehicle for achieving the new deep voice and we would work on that until he was successful. Often it was very tough going, but gradually Phil began to be able even to read aloud what he had written without losing his voice or going into the falsetto, and finally he was even able to talk to others with some ease. I almost became a substitute father of sorts, certainly a forgiving one. The fire was an accident. It had happened long ago. It was time to look forward, not backward. He had a life to live. I got him a part-time job and enlisted the aid of some pretty female graduate students to enlarge his social contacts while still monitoring his voice. Within four months Phil was symptom-free and a different person. Life was very good.

Too good! Suddenly one day Phil showed up with the worst case of acne I have ever seen. It covered his face, neck and even his hands. He was sent to the Health Service but to no avail; nothing seemed to help. Week after week the acne persisted and the better he spoke the worse it became. I was appalled. What had gone wrong? Certainly the well-known conversion reaction had occurred, but was he not worse off than when he first came to the clinic? I had created a visual monster. He was repulsive!

At first, Phil did not seem to share my misgivings. Indeed, he seemed strangely indifferent to his blotched appearance. He was now able to talk; he would outgrow the acne, he said. But later, as it continued to spread over his body and into his scalp instead of disappearing, Phil began again to be withdrawn and moody. I began to hear a few tiny pitch breaks.

It seemed obvious that the underlying guilt had not been dissipated, despite all the work we had done for so many months. Absolution, forgiveness were not enough. I went to Phil's pastor for help. He was sympathetic and understanding but told me that much as he valued and prized the role of religious experience in such matters, he doubted that Philip would ever find surcease that way. He had tried; Philip had tried. They had prayed together for forgiveness and absolution. A tragedy! Perhaps the boy would have to pay a penance of some sort. These things happened. The pastor was discouraged and discouraging.

One day I had the occasion to do a little drinking with some physician friends of mine and of course heard the usual medical shop talk. When it happened to turn to acne I described what had happened to Phil and asked if they knew of any new treatment for it. One of them, a dermatologist, proposed that I refer the young man to him. "I'd like to try out something I've read about—flaying. A lot of reports have been coming out recommending it. It seems that by using a sun lamp you first burn the skin, then carefully and repeatedly scrape off the epidermal layers. As the new skin is formed, the acne disappears." Flaying! Penance?

When I told Phil about it, his eyes gleamed with interest and he accepted the suggestion immediately. I could just read what was going on behind that pocked, blotched, scaly red face of his. "Hurt me! Flay me! Burn me! Good!" Poor devil. The treatment lasted several months, and during this period his speech was perfect. No moments of muteness; no pitch breaks; no falsetto. A fine deep bass voice. He could talk that way anywhere, any time, to anyone. On the days after he was burned, his face was a mess but he wore bandages over it only because the physician insisted, preferring to show that burned face to the world. Whenever it had healed sufficiently to permit some more scraping, he was happier than I had ever known him to be. Smiling and laughing, he would tell me how much it hurt to be flayed. Was he paying for his sin and finding relief from guilt—knowing at last the peace that passeth understanding? Sometimes he reminded me of an old renegade I had known in my youth who dearly loved to confess and get religion. At the first news that some evangelist would be coming to town, Old Man McGee would hurry to collect some sins so he could publicly confess them up there at the pulpit with great lamentations and expressions of penitence. The nobility and serenity on his face afterward impressed me greatly. Much more than his sins! Anyway, Phil wore Old Man McGee's look.

Finally Phil's treatment ended and he had a new face, pink as a baby's, though a bit scarred around the edges. I bought him a mirror and told him to look at himself ten times a day and to remember how much he had suffered and to tell himself he had suffered enough. And to use his bass voice while doing so!

For two months Phil was fine. He now was thinking about going into some field of human service, perhaps even becoming a preacher. He wanted to help other people in trouble. Perhaps he should join the Salvation Army. Or become a missionary? Or a doctor? Each week it was something different. Toward the end of this period he mentioned (and I noticed) that some miniature pitch breaks were coming back into his voice. Gad, I thought, here we go again!

For several more months we wrestled with Phil's demon as his old behaviors came back, first the pitch breaks, then the falsetto, and finally even moments of not being able to phonate. The acne, however, had not returned. It was his voice now that concerned him. Everything we tried seemed to be of no avail; he just got worse and worse, though he never got as bad as he had been when he first came. He began to write long papers about his miseries. Into me he flushed his evil feelings toward self so often I thought of terminating our relationship but when I remembered his pantomimed, "Help me! Help me if you can!" I couldn't refuse.

Then suddenly Phil recovered. The voice was as good or better than it had ever been. He was untroubled, very happy. He had decided to become a teacher after all. What had happened? He didn't know. This happened during his last year of college. A school superintendent of a small town school system had interviewed Phil and was so impressed that he gave him a contract for the following year as a high school teacher of social studies. All was well! I crossed my eyes, fingers, and legs superstitiously and waited.

He began to see me infrequently. Didn't need me any more, he said. He was doing fine. His aunt wrote me a letter of appreciation. His pastor called to say that Philip had evidently finally made his peace with God and had received forgiveness for that unfortunate happening so long ago. I waited and I worried. Such miracles do not occur in Kalamazoo.

I did not have to wait long. One day I received two phone calls that provided the explanation. The first was from Phil's academic counselor who had just learned that he was flunking every one of his college courses, that he had not turned in a single assignment, and had absented himself from class far too frequently. He probably wouldn't be able to graduate unless he shaped up immediately. The other call came from the dean of men. Phil had been caught in the act of stealing a silver service from his dormitory housemother's room. He was in deep trouble. Two new hooks on which to hang his guilt and himself.

I was tempted to do nothing at all. Lord, hadn't I done enough? Surely my role as a speech pathologist had been accomplished. Phil had his male voice. If I intervened in his morbid quest for self-punishment, wouldn't I just make matters worse again? Let the poor devil suffer! Let him feed upon his guilt, bathe in it. Why should I get involved again?

But I couldn't play Pontius Pilate and wash my hands, so I went to the dean and each of Phil's instructors, violated my oath of confidentiality, and told them his story. I made quite a presentation about the need for time gaining and working through conflicts, about his struggles and how he had conquered his voice problems and acne, and convinced the dean that punishing Phil would only feed his guilt, not diminish it. His instructors were reminded that flunking Phil would scratch the only chance he had to begin a new life in a position of respect as a high school teacher. I would take all the responsibility, but please give him a chance. The intervention must have been pretty eloquent because I learned later that one of them had given Phil an A in his course (which made *me* feel a bit guilty). Anyway, he graduated and didn't go to jail.

But before he left we had one final conference in which we reviewed the entire history of the problem. Phil was able to verbalize fairly objectively the dynamics of what had taken place. He showed considerable insight about the relationship of his guilt feelings to his voice problem, his acne, and other behaviors. He said that he had decided to bury the past, that it had bedeviled him long enough. He now had a chance to live a new life and intended to do so. It was good to hear him speaking so well and so hopefully. Perhaps at last he had slain his dragon. It sounded too good to be true. Besides, I remembered earlier conferences when Phil had mentioned occasional thoughts of suicide. Would that be his final solution or absolution?

Uncharacteristically, no attempt was made to contact Phil during the next year or two, nor did he contact us. Then one day a phone call came from his aunt asking for an immediate appointment. She had something very important

to discuss discreetly with me. No, he wasn't dead. He had been very successful as a teacher. His speech was fine. No more acne. He had been in no
trouble whatsoever. It was just. . . .

When she showed up, Phil's aunt had great difficulty in coming to the
point. She corroborated again the information she had given me about how
splendidly Phil was doing on the job. She did say that he was still thinking
about becoming a preacher and had been working with derelicts in the mis-
sions of a slum area in a nearby city. Finally, I had to ask her bluntly what she
wanted to discuss and she hesitantly told me. Phil had just brought home his
bride-to-be. Her name was Mame and she was at least twenty years older than
Philip and. . . . Again the aunt fumbled for words. "It's just . . . It's just that
she . . . It's bad enough that she's so much older but . . . Oh, Doctor, I've
learned that she . . . that she was a prostitute."

I have followed up that marriage ever since. They have lived happily
ever after. They really have. Perhaps you can explain why.

In olden times, when a deviant was viewed as a threat to society, he was
given a stigma. Thieves were branded on the forehead with the letter T, or had a
hand cut off. Lepers had to wear distinctive clothing and, by chanting constantly,
warn others that they had the disease. Women who performed adultery had the
scarlet letter A emblazoned with fire upon their breasts. We do not do these
things today, but the deviant is stigmatized nevertheless. Sometimes we find in
the abnormal speech behavior itself the stigma, the symbol of guilt.

Vicky was sent to me by a parish priest (who had known her since
childhood) because she had started to stutter shortly after her nineteenth
birthday and was getting worse. She was probably the most miserable, dirty,
bedraggled, scared young woman I have ever seen. A mess. "I don't know
what's wrong with her," the priest had said over the phone, "but every time
she tries to talk, her mouth just freezes and then she snorts." His picture was
pretty accurate but what impressed me most was the message of her body
English which seemed to say to me "I am frightened. I must be careful and
guarded. I am in danger."

We worked very gently with Vicky and very slowly, almost obliquely,
for when stuttering suddenly appears in adulthood in a monosymptomatic
form it often has been precipitated by some severe emotional trauma. Indeed,
my plan was to offer only a token, supportive therapy until she could be
referred to a psychiatrist friend in whom I had confidence. I concentrated on
helping her to get phonation started, on reinforcing the fluency she did possess, and above all, on trying to get her to trust another person. No attempt
was made to probe her past experiences. I would let her tell me when she was
ready. Often I wanted to suggest that Vicky at least take a bath or comb her
hair, but I didn't, even though my office stank for minutes after she left. After

many sessions it became apparent that some real rapport (whatever that means) had been achieved. Vicky's face had lost its panicky expression and she no longer held herself so rigidly. She began to confide little bits of self-revelation that I mildly discouraged. Then, perhaps, I made a mistake. I began to try to modify the sniffing and snorting which she had been using to terminate the long laryngeal fixations. Nothing happened. Vicky refused to confront these behaviors or to modify them, or even to try to do so. I should have known better, but once when her resistance was dramatically evident I suddenly asked her what she was smelling when she sniffed.

All hell broke loose. The boil had been lanced. The dam had been breeched. Pandora's box had been opened. Vicky cried and cursed me and flung herself out of her chair. "Semen!" she screamed. "That's what I smell and what I smell of—SEMEN!" And she ran from the room.

Some days passed before I saw Vicky again, but finally she came back and finally she told me all the story, a sad one. When her mother had died suddenly, her father was inconsolable. The family had been very close and loving. He grieved and grieved, wouldn't even go to work, just mourned. Then one night when Vicky heard him sobbing in his bed, she went into it to comfort him and you can guess the rest. She said that her "stuttering" had started when she went to confession. Well, I persuaded her to go to the priest, separated her from the old goat, enrolled her in college where she lived in the dorm, found her some boy friends, continued to support her during her penance and travail by going through the motions of speech therapy. As the whole tangled mess unravelled, her stuttering disappeared completely and she became a clean, well-groomed, very attractive person.

Many years later I met Vicky downtown, a very well-dressed mature woman. I'm sure she must have seen me coming for quite a distance, but she looked through me without a sign of recognition as she passed. And I, of course, reciprocated. Two strangers passing by. I'm sorry to have to confess, though, that I permitted myself, some paces beyond that confrontation, one very small, short sniff.

the psychotic client

We now turn to the problems of those who respond to an unbearable reality by distorting it—the psychotics who create their own worlds. Not many of them will come your way, but when they do, you must be able to recognize them and to make the proper referrals. Several authors have claimed that very, very few stutterers are psychotic and those who become psychotic lose their stuttering immediately. I have never counted the stutterers with whom I've worked intensively but there have been a large number of them. Yet in all that host I can recall only four who could be called truly psychotic. Since all of them are now institutionalized, deteriorated or dead, here are their clinical pictures.

The first one was Boris, a tiny gnome of a tailor, about forty years old. He had come to this country from Bulgaria in his youth and he specialized in tailoring furs, as we discovered when the nurses in our health service complained that Boris would follow them around the corridors ogling them lasciviously. No, said Boris, he hated women; he was just mentally measuring them for the fur coats he might design for them. During our group meetings, Boris was far away from any human contact. He said nothing, just looked into space blankly. Individual sessions with him, however, were very lively. He told me how I should cure him, that I must divulge to him the magic word that would free his tongue. Some soothsayer in Bulgaria had once informed him that this would happen in a faraway country. I told him I didn't know the word but I would help him find it if he would do some other things first—the activities of our regular therapy. He agreed and did whatever I asked so long as each session would conclude with some search for the word. It had three syllables, Boris said, and began with the letter D. I entered into his delusions as best I could under the guidance of a psychiatrist friend who said he was interested but not interested enough to take Boris on as a patient.

After the little tailor had come to trust me, he told me that he was not one person but two. The other one, the invisible one, was bad but didn't stutter because he knew the word and wouldn't tell Boris. *He* was *right there,* Boris said, pointing over his left shoulder. I even got so I could talk to his alter ego at times, and when Boris responded in that role he was indeed completely fluent. His deep bass voice then was quite unlike his habitual one, so I could generally know in our three-way conversation who was speaking to whom, though there were a few times when I got confused. One of these times made Boris' other self furious and he and Boris had quite a discussion over whether I should be killed for my stupidity, but Boris won the argument. "No," he said, "the little Doc is a nice man. Yah, he's not too bright but he's trying to help me find my word. No, I'm not going to kill him. No!" I wondered how the little tailor (I was a foot taller than he was) would commit the mayhem— with a needle or the scissors? I had worked with him and "his friend" for three months when suddenly Boris disappeared and I have not seen nor heard from him since. All I have is a yellowed scrap of paper saying, "Thanks. I've found my word." A shame Boris didn't share it. I could then go back to my birch tree and say I'd fulfilled the oath of my youth that someday I'd find the cure for stuttering. Let's see . . . "Daskalov, no, . . . Dobrovitch . . . no . . . ."

Another stutterer with hallucinations has plagued me and several other so-called authorities in the field of stuttering for many years. Let us call him Hal. Hal writes letters to us often, for he is convinced that he has found the cure for stuttering and he cannot understand why we fail to welcome it with open arms. My file of his letters is two inches thick, but his theme is usually the same. It is this: whenever a stutterer stutters, the whole world must rise up and stutter back at him. Hal believes in aversive stimulation and contingencies. I provide a typical and verbatim sample of our one-sided correspondence:

"I am but a live human body, and I need not report the experience here, but, I am also a scientisft, therefore, I must report my expcrience to you and some of the other researchists on stuttering. In 1954, I was reading Glasner's arficle discribing how they attempted to set up a system in Baltimorfe to cure all of that city's stutterers. At that time, I experience a nerve excitation in my brain. that is, it was a physical occurrence. the nerves of my brain activafed. This had never occurred before this date. Since that time until the present, only when I think of relafionships of curing stutters, does, this excitation of the Brain nerves occurr. I have a monomania on thfe problem of stuttering somewhat like Wendell Johnson had. although I will be doing something elas I unconcouiously be thinking about the problem of stuttering. This is a physical thing since thfe brain nerves excite on thought of stuttering cure for 15 million stutters, how tb do it, proof of mthod etc."

"In, 1959, I began to derive meaning from thunder sound. Some people believe thunder sound to man meaning is communication with God or dead souls. Since 1959, I have only been hit with about 10 meaning. Examples of this meaning are 'Come', 'Jesus Christ is Here' 'Get marryd', 'Stutter at Stutterer' I believe this to be a physical thing. The crach or sound of thunder will not sound of my own mind. On a couple of occations, I had to be thinking about a train of thought related to what the thunder sound expressed, but the sound meaning may come out of nothing that I was thinking about. On one occation I remember, that I was researching in library a subject and a direction meaning came to me from thunder sound because I was researching that matter. I believe this thunder sound to me communication is relevant to the problem of stuttering, because I am a stutter only because the whole world will not stutter back at me with a thunder.''

Hal attended our clinic for two weeks one spring, during which time I tried my utmost to get him psychiatric help—even unto offering to pay for it myself. Hal refused. He wasn't crazy. I was—and all the other speech pathologists in the world were too. The solution to the problem of stuttering was so obvious. Why couldn't I see its logic? He didn't want any speech therapy either; he just wanted to persuade me. After he left, he wrote that he was very disappointed in me but would now contact Joseph Sheehan, Wendell Johnson and others who would have more sense.

I only saw Hal once thereafter. It was late evening one fall day when a masked man tapped on the window of our old farm house and shouted that I should open the door. With my shotgun in hand I did so, and there was Hal. "I have The Answer," he intoned, "for I am a P-p-p-p-prophet!" "So you are," I said. "I'll see you tomorrow at the office and you can tell me all about it." Hal refused. "My vision is on me now," he insisted, "and I must tell you now." He tried to force his way into the house but I pushed him out and locked the door, saying again that I'd see him in the morning. I watched him walk down the lane in the bitter cold and felt badly enough after a few minutes to get into my car to give him a ride back to town. But he refused, cursing me when I stopped him. "Fifteen million stutterers and you turn me away. May they haunt you, old fool!" were his final words. From a colleague I learned that Hal is now in prison—"just for causing a small one-inch scar"—but he still seeks to persuade someone to help him solve the problem of stuttering. Just like me!

These first two clients I considered relatively harmless; the third, Carl, was not. My first encounter with him took place on the stairs to my office, where I was hurrying to keep an appointment with some stutterer who had written me from an army camp in Texas. At the top step, a man accosted me furiously and demanded to know why I was following him. Since he was in uniform, I introduced myself, explained that I was late, and sorry, and that I was glad to have arrived at the same time he did. He asked me several times if I were indeed Dr. Van Riper, but only after my secretary greeted me by name did he seem to calm down.

Our interview soon revealed Carl's paranoia. Other people made him stutter; they had it in for him. They had put him in the army and he wanted out. Carl asked if his commanding officer had written me and he pawed through my mail on the desk even after my secretary had responded to my query negatively. Yes, he wanted to get rid of his stuttering, but the only way that could be done was by "taking care" of the enemies "who had put it on" him in the first place. One of them was a Baptist preacher. Did I know him? Had he ever written me? Was I sure?

Carl's stuttering, like most of the other of these odd ones, was mild—primarily consisting of many syllabic repetitions, never any complete blocking nor any signs of avoidance, postponement or struggle. His eye contact was excellent—almost hypnotic. Every so often Carl would suddenly become very angry with me about something I had asked. For example, he glared at me murderously when I began to delve into his family history. All in all, it was a most unsatisfactory examination session that ended only when he gave me the name of his commanding officer and ordered me to write him requesting his immediate discharge.

After some soul-searching, I decided not to honor his demand and forgot all about him until about a year later when I received a phone call from Atlanta. It was Carl. He was out of the army at last, he said. No thanks to me. He knew I'd written his officer to put him in the hospital under guard and to give him shock treatment "Well," he said, "you'll never do it to another stutterer." Carl said he was going to kill me. "I'll be seeing you, Doc," he said. "Take care!"

That next week provided a series of phone calls from Carl, each with the same threat, and each from a city a bit closer to Kalamazoo. Then I had a phone call from a woman who said she ran a rooming house for transients and that a man who talked crazy-like told her he was going up to the college to shoot him a Professor Van Riper. She said he had something in his pocket that bulged like a pistol. So I called the chief of police, who pooh-poohed the whole thing. "Hell, he hasn't done anything yet, has he? If we arrested every bird who made threats we'd have to use the schoolhouses for jails. If you find he has a gun on him, we'll send a man up. Just call us."

So I went to the clinic lab, got a small crowbar we'd used to open boxes, and had a student, now head of a Department of Communication Disorders in one of the mountain states, rehearse the act of hitting an imaginary man over the head when I gave a signal. I was hoping that our hurried rehearsal had been sufficient when my secretary called to say there was a man to see me. As she ushered Carl in, I couldn't help but look and yes, there was indeed a bulge in his side pocket. Surprisingly, he seemed to be in an excellent mood and wanted to talk. Perhaps the cat playing with the mouse, I thought, but I went along with the conversation. Then I had an inspiration. I told Carl that I had described his problem to a doctor friend of mine who had expressed a real desire to see him and that I'd sure like to have a report of his findings before beginning the stuttering therapy. Carl seemed pleased and interested, so I called a psychiatrist and made an appointment for that afternoon. Late in the evening the psychiatrist called me at home to say that he had examined my patient, that Carl was a bit schizoid but harmless, and that he would see him a few more times before sending him on his way. I tried to tell him about the threats I'd received and the evidences of paranoia I'd discovered, but he just laughed. "He's harmless. Quit worrying. He's not the kind to do anything."

The next morning when Carl arrived, my student was again in the office adjacent to mine, the door was open, and we had rehearsed a bit more. It was fortunate, for Carl was very surly that morning. Yes, he'd seen the doctor and he didn't think much of him, though he'd go back that afternoon for one more examination. The conversation was very strained and unproductive and his hand kept straying toward his side pocket. Finally, as he got up to leave, he patted that pocket and said, "I give you one more day to live, Doc. I know your game."

So I called up the psychiatrist and lied. "Carl has just been here and I thought I ought to warn you. I think he has a gun in his pocket and he told me that he's going to kill me tomorrow but that first he'll kill you this afternoon." I never saw Carl again. The psychiatrist had him in the back ward of our state hospital for the insane before nightfall. My former student should know that I still have that crowbar in my office.

The last of my handful I shall call Josie. She was a tall, angular female of uncertain age who had been referred to us by a certain midwestern university clinic. I always resented it a bit that they failed to inform me that Josie also had previously been a patient in a mental hospital there for two years. For most of the year Josie was fairly sane, if a little bizarre, and it was fortunate that therapy was initiated with her in the fall, for every spring she went off the deep end into a real psychotic episode. Our therapy was very easy and very successful. By Christmas Josie was entirely fluent in all situations and under all conditions. She stayed that way until the first blossoms of May, when she relapsed badly—a pattern that repeated itself for the six years that I followed her case and until she moved out of our vicinity. Each time she relapsed Josie had a new hang-up to accompany her renewed stuttering. I shall tell you only about the two final ones.

Josie appeared again at the clinic on the second of May that year after scaring my wife with a visit to my home while I was on a trip. "You are a fortunate woman, Mrs. Van Riper," she said in the hollow lugubrious monotone she often used when her stuttering was bad. "You have a lovely young daughter and I have none. You have a brilliant husband and I have none. Do you think that is fair?" Her long silences and piercing gaze were hard to bear. Anyway, that year Josie asked me for five hundred dollars. "You see, Dr. Van Riper, it cost me that much to go to the other university. Now that you've c-c-cured me, I'd like to have the money back, please."

OUR CLIENTS **59**

Every session we had with Josie ended with the same request and there were times when I contemplated paying the ransom if she would only let me alone. But June came at last and Josie was fluent enough again to go her way.

I could tell many tales about Josie but will content myself with the one about her final appearance the following Maytime. In she walked, as gaunt and awkward as ever, sat herself down not across the desk but to one side and fixed her piercing gaze on what I thought was my belt buckle. She never looked directly at my face in all of our interview as I made arrangements for another booster session to tide her over the pangs of springtime. Finally I asked her why she didn't look at me and she replied, "Dr. Van Riper, as you well know, you have given me a compulsion and a complex in exchange for my stuttering. I now cannot take my eyes off the fly of a male's pair of pants. My eyes are glued to his crotch, sir, and I cannot remove them. I would appreciate it, sir, if you would take away this curse."

So I did. I told her that the only way to get rid of it was to fake some highly voluntary stuttering and that every time she found herself fixating with her eyes, or having some involuntary stuttering, she should do that pseudo-stuttering very deliberately. Lo and behold, the formula worked! Within a week she no longer had to look at male bifurcations nor to stutter. She was very fluent and free as she came gratefully to tell me that she had a new job in the hospital as a lab technician and no longer needed my services. "Also," she said, "I have a new hobby. I've taken up fencing."

Hurriedly I crossed my legs.

These four stutterers, together with other psychotic clients with different disorders, reflect, as in a dark mirror, the tragi-comic aspect of all humankind. They taught me that their aberrations were universal, that all of us delude ourselves, that all of us at times distort reality. On sanity's yardstick (an elastic one) we oscillate up and down, if not with the seasons, then certainly under certain conditions of stress. We all have experienced unfounded suspicions. Yes, we're all a little mad. Beginning clinicians often expect their clients to behave rationally, but reason, sweet reason, is not a very effective clinical tool. We just are not very rational creatures. If we were, there would be no poets—or clinicians. So here's to madness, especially in the spring.

DIAGNOSTIC PROBLEMS

Student clinicians always get a real charge from participating in their first diagnostic examination. At long last they are becoming professional. They have had their basic courses. They have become acquainted with the various standardized tests and have been trained to observe and evaluate the human behaviors that constitute our field of endeavor. At last it is time for them to come to the aid of the party. They respond with a blend of excited anticipation and uneasiness.

Nature of the Deviancy

There are a few tales to tell that may justify that uneasiness. The diagnostic process is not always an easy one. Even its first question: "What's wrong with this client's speech and language?" can contain its boobytraps.

I remember well a Mrs. Green, a farmer's wife, not very bright, who was given an appointment to have us examine her stuttering son. As is my custom, I saw her first to get some overview of the problem. "Mrs. Green, I understand that your boy Willy stutters." She nodded. "Can you describe to me just what he does when he stutters?" She told me enough to convince me that Willy really had a severe problem. Then she was asked how Willy felt about his stuttering and how his brothers and sisters or playmates reacted to it. Again, she provided enough illustrative material to indicate that the boy had been penalized frequently and had developed fear and shame responses. So I thanked her and went down to see the boy who had been waiting in the playroom.

Well, I worked with that boy for over an hour and did not find any trace of stuttering. When he was queried about the subject of being mocked by the other kids about his stuttering, he denied that they had ever teased him about it. I put him in various stress situations. Again, no stuttering. Finally I went back to see his mother.

"Mrs. Green," I said, "I'm sorry but I fear I cannot help you—because I was unable to get enough of a sample of your boy's stuttering to analyze it." She began to say something but I continued. "Stuttering is a curious disorder, Mrs. Green, because sometimes under certain conditions the person will be perfectly fluent." On and on I went, explaining, justifying my failure to find Willy's stuttering, until finally she interrupted me. "Oh, that's Johnny, not Willy. Willy wuz sick today so I brung his brudder for company." Gad!

Then there was James, referred to us by his public school clinician. He lalled, the clinician told us in her letter, and "perhaps he has some apraxia." James seemed to be able to raise the tip of his tongue, to dot the palate with it fairly swiftly, and "even to lick the bottom of his nose," but when he spoke, he kept the tongue flat in the mouth, and many sounds were distorted. She said that James had become very sensitive about his speech problem and was refusing to recite in school. Because both parents worked days, the clinician would bring him to the clinic.

While I interviewed my public school colleague, I had one of my better graduate students administer several standardized articulation tests to the boy. The report was very detailed, with all the errors duly noted and classified. Much inconsistency. James could produce every phoneme perfectly in isolation or nonsense syllables. Responded poorly to trial therapy. Possibility of apraxia.

Getting some oral stereognosis forms from the cupboard, I went down to see the boy, and as usual, conversed with him for a few moments. Hell, James was not apraxic at all. He was a stutterer who was using a lalling kind of speaking to provide him with a precarious fluency. Many stutterers can be temporarily fluent when assuming a strange way of talking. The boy admitted that "it didn't always work" and that was why he wouldn't try to recite in school.

Then there was Mary, a college student whose voice was so monopitched and without inflection that she was refused entrance into the teaching curriculum. In my first contact, I had time to get just a cursory impression. A dead voice, so monotonous she sounded like a robot talking. Mary also presented the picture of always being on guard. Her postures were rigid and fixed; there were practically no hand gestures. Her face was blank and without expression, almost a mask, as she told me she had been seen at the counseling center. So I told Mary I would see her again after I got the center's report, if she would give me permission to have this information. She signed the blank without any resistance. "I'm OK," she said. "It's just my voice." The counseling center's report said the same thing.

When we met again, I gave her a very comprehensive voice examination, verbalizing my findings as we proceeded, showing my interest, and I hope competence, and soon the whole strange story came out. Mary had been using the monopitch to keep from showing the pitch breaks and diplophonia which were her real problem and concern. It was the only way she could talk without having her voice flipflop around or having that odd fluttering in it. When I asked her to stop guarding herself and to speak spontaneously, she finally managed to do so. It was then easy to understand her need for the monopitch. Unlike most pitch breaks, Mary's suddenly broke downward, not upward into any falsetto, and the downward shift was about an octave or even more. A very abnormal sounding voice! It was easy to understand why she would try to prevent these breaks from happening if she could. But I also heard other strange features. Mixed in with the pitch breaks were bits of a deep bass voice! I could hardly believe my ears. A man's bass voice coming out of the mouth of that very feminine girl? It was impossible. Fortunately, I had been recording our sessions and so I played it back to make sure I wasn't having hallucinations. No, those little segments were keyed about a pitch level of almost two octaves below Middle C. I have a deep voice and when I tried to hum and match the pitch level, I found it at the very bottom of my own range. Still incredulous, I looked up to find Mary grinning like a Chessie Cat.

"Yes," she said, "I can talk like that any time. Listen." She proceeded to do so. When I shut my eyes, I would have sworn that the voice was coming from the low man in a barbershop quartet.

Mary said that she had discovered how to use the low voice during her early teens, and had used it "for kicks" to amuse herself and others. She told how she had scared her roommate in college by suddenly commanding her in that deep man's voice to take off her clothes and get into bed immediately. It had been a real asset at parties. Mary also stated and demonstrated that she could alternate between her high natural voice and the deep voice at will, and use both voices simultaneously when singing to harmonize with herself.

The harmony wasn't very good, always having a fixed interval between the two pitches, but it was there. Sounded like a man and woman having a lousy duet. Mary had even thought of exploiting her unusual voices and going into show business, as many of her friends had suggested, but then, she said, she began to lose control. If she used the bass voice very long, she found it difficult to shift back to her own. Gradually, when the pitch breaks began to appear involuntarily along with moments of the double voice, she became terrified. After several very traumatic situations, she had hunted frantically for some way of preventing the breaks and found that she could do so by speaking in a monopitch. What happened then, of course, was that a fear of speaking rapidly developed. "I began to think I couldn't talk at all without that crutch," Mary told me. She had often tried to go back to her own natural voice, but the more she used it the more fear she had that it would shift or wobble or be the deep bass voice. She begged for help.

I was able to give it. I had noticed that when Mary used the bass voice, she assumed an odd head posture for vocalization. She cocked her head forward, but lowered her chin and tensed her neck muscles. She also exhaled deeply and then vocalized on the complemental air that remained. None of these behaviors occurred when she used either her own high voice or the monopitch. With some desensitization, negative practice, and positive reinforcement for the normal vocal postures, Mary solved her problem. I still have the tape recording.

During the last fifty years, the terms used to designate the workers of our professional vineyard have changed from *speech correctionist* and *speech therapist* to the current ones of speech and language clinician or speech pathologist. Many years ago, Martin Palmer and others tried hard but unsuccessfully to baptize us with the name *logopedist* after the European usage, and more recently the terms communicologist, spaudologist and other verbal monstrosities have been suggested but have failed to gain acceptance. Personally, I never cared what they called me so long as I could help untangle tongues and lives.

Similarly, marked changes have occurred in the treatment of individuals with speech disorders. When I began to practice, more than forty years ago, the mental hygiene movement was in its heydey and most speech problems were viewed as either organic in nature or due to emotional conflicts. Stuttering was regarded as a neurosis; so was dysphonia. Misarticulations were termed "infantile perseverations," and were to be treated by psychoanalyzing the client or his parents, by cutting the client's frenum, or by using tongue and breathing exercises. The person with aphasia was untreatable.

But fashions have changed and they will change again. Currently, most of our clients are seen by many workers as simply possessing a learning problem. Their communication difficulties are considered the result of bad habits. Through behavior modification procedures—especially those based upon operant conditioning—acceptable new responses can be instated, reinforced, and the old ones extinguished. The emphasis is upon observable behaviors that can be counted, upon reinforcers that can be made contingent. Etiology is eliminated as of no concern. The question is *what,* not *why.*

Reasons for the Deviant Behavior

Nevertheless, there are times when a clinician should ask "*Why?*" There are clients whose antecedent events as revealed by the case history are very important to the design of therapy. So it was with Teddy.

Teddy's clinician, new to the field and thoroughly trained in operant conditioning, came to ask my help. "I work in the public schools," she said, "and I have a boy, the son of the superintendent, whom I haven't been able to help at all. Nor could my predecessor, who was fired because she couldn't help him either. His name is Teddy and he's about to have his ninth birthday. Very bright too. Reads above his grade level and does well in school, but his spontaneous speech is almost unintelligible. Even his parents have trouble understanding him. Now, what's strange is that he can make every sound perfectly in syllables and in short words when repeating them after me, but he can't prolong them at all in isolation and he makes strange errors every time he uses connected speech. I just can't get any carry-over at all. The moment he uses polysyllabic words or strings words together he becomes almost completely unintelligible."

I asked her how she had been treating Teddy, and she brought out her operant programs, complete with baselines, objectives, criteria, and schedules of reinforcement. Very impressive, but she said they hadn't worked. "I've done everything I know to get Teddy to combine those perfectly spoken words into phrases and sentences, but I've failed. I've varied the steps and the reinforcements, but I just can't get any transfer. Let me play this cassette for you."

It showed clearly that what she had told me was true. Teddy was indeed able to produce all the speech sounds perfectly, except he could not prolong them *in isolation*. He could even say them perfectly when reading syllables or short words without her stimulation. But when he had to read a whole sentence, or speak spontaneously, a whole host of errors appeared and what he said could not be understood. On one part of the tape, Teddy first said each of these words correctly: *the, girl, likes, to, go, to, the, store;* and then, when he read the same words in a complete sentence, the utterance was incomprehensible.

Moreover, Teddy's misarticulation errors were not the usual ones. He substituted the /h/ for the /θ/ or /ʒ/; the /f/ for the /t/ and /d/, and the /k/ and /g/; the /l/ for the /n/. He even had trouble with the /b/ and /m/ sounds, using a distorted /v/ as their replacement. And there were omissions of final sounds and very unusual errors. The therapist grinned. "I told you Teddy was different from the ordinary garden variety of articulation case. His mistakes are random. Why does he even have trouble saying the /m/ or /b/? Why in the world does he substitute an /l/ for an /n/? The other day I heard him first say *rare* for *chair* and later on, *lair* for the same word. They make no sense."

"Behavior is never random," I replied, "and there's always sense in nonsense, as Alice in Wonderland clearly showed. In fact, just by analyzing the errors in that small sample, I've got a pretty good idea of what's wrong and what should be done."

She was skeptical and sarcastic. "OK, Sherlock Holmes. I'm your Mz. Watson. What do you deduce, sir?" For the hell of it, though I was far from certain about the guesses I had made, I decided to play the role.

"All right, Mz. Watson," I said. "If you will interview Teddy's parents and get a complete case history, which I understand you have not done, you will find that Teddy is so afraid of the water he will not learn to swim, and that he always sleeps with his arms outside the covers and snores loudly. Moreover, he will drink milk at home but not in school. And when he is given an all day sucker, the kind with a stick, he only licks it and will never suck it. He also has had frequent earaches."

My public school colleague was incredulous. "Mr. Holmes, you are a monstrous fraud but I'll check to make sure," she said. "How can you come up with all that nonsense from merely hearing a little sample of Teddy's speech?"

"Elementary, Mz. Watson. Elementary," I replied. "Those deductions are obvious but let me write down some others and seal them in this envelope. We'll open it after you've been able to interview the parents. Also, please examine the boy's mouth, throat, and nose. Then we'll have a conference and I'll see Teddy and outline what might be done."

This is what I wrote and sealed in the envelope: "A blue baby due to anoxia at birth? A history of asthma or hay fever or other allergies? Nasal polyps or deviated nasal septum? Adenoids or adenectomy? A history of apnea?"

When we met again, Teddy was sick and couldn't come. "Mr. Holmes," the therapist said, "you were right on all but one count: Teddy does not snore loudly. He does sleep always on his back, and with his arms outside the covers, and how did you know that? He has also had a lot of earaches. He does lick the sucker and won't put it into his mouth. His parents said he was deathly afraid of the water. And I just can't believe it, Sherlock, but you were even right about the milk. I talked to his teacher and she says he won't touch it, but his parents insisted that he regularly drank it at home. How in the world did you ever know these things just from listening to a short tape?"

"Elementary, Mz. Watson. The milk at school is always served in cartons and he would have to drink it through a straw. At home he drinks it from a cup or glass. Of course he would have those odd articulation errors." As I handed her the envelop to open, I read her report of the case history she had taken.

"Oh, oh," she exclaimed. "I didn't explore the birth history, but what's being a blue baby got to do with Teddy's articulation problem? Yes, the mother told me he had been under medication for asthma for several years but now seems to have outgrown the problem. No hay fever or allergies, though. And he had his adenoids removed along with his tonsils last year. The doctor told her they were the worst he had ever seen in an eight-year-old child. Gave her the devil for not having them out earlier. As for nasal polyps, I could see none when I examined the boy. Maybe they're further back. He does have a deviated septum. Couldn't blow out of the left nostril at all. But the right passageway seems to be OK. What's apnea? I never heard of it."

"A transient difficulty in being able to breathe," I told her. "It can be pretty scary for a child, or for that matter for an adult too, especially when it occurs in one's sleep. Does Teddy have trouble sleeping?"

"Well, his mother said he has always had frequent nightmares." My colleague was upset. "Let's quit this Sherlock Holmes stuff, please," she begged. "I'm all mixed up and confused. Level with me. How does all this stuff fit together?"

I relented. "My basic hypothesis is that Teddy is afraid of occluding his oral airway," I explained. "Afraid that if he does, he can't breathe. He tries to talk without ever blocking it—even for an instant. That's pretty far-fetched, I suppose, but let's review our findings. First of all, Teddy uses fricative sounds instead of the plosives. Why? Secondly, he substitutes the usually difficult /r/ and /l/ for the usually easy /m/ and /n/ nasals. Why? Nasal sounds block the oral passageway, so he won't use them. Thirdly, although you have been able to get Teddy to make every sound correctly in syllables and monosyllabic words, he cannot (or will not) try to prolong them in isolation—which would take a longer exhalation. Longer words, and phrases and sentences also take longer exhalation times, and the only way Teddy can be sure that his oral airway is always open is to use a kind of articulation that never blocks it. That's why he uses the /f/ and /v/ for all stop consonants and the /r/ and /l/ as replacements. He thinks he has to keep that airway open and he'll use no sound that plugs it. And that's why he won't say the easy /m/, /n/ or /p/ and /b/ sounds. I noticed, too, on the tape that every time he said one of those syllables or single words correctly, he uttered it on one breath. Even when he counted, each number was spoken separately on a single exhalation. I also could hear him inhale between each word or syllable—which probably meant that he was a mouth breather."

"Yes, he is," she interrupted, "I've noticed that too. But I found no evidence of a tongue thrust habit or reverse swallow. Do you think the mouth breathing was due to the adenoids?"

"Who knows?" I answered. "It could have been that, or to the asthma perhaps. If he had earaches, the nasal passages and Eustachian tube could have been pretty well blocked for some time, so it was probably the adenoids and not the septum that prevented Teddy from breathing through his nose. When you combine an inability to inhale through the nose with the breath hunger of asthma, the need for an open airway through the mouth can be terribly important to a child. Perhaps he does have some apnea, though I'd consider that explanation almost as far out and unconvincing as attributing the problem to imprinting at birth—the anoxia bit.

"Actually, I haven't the slightest bit of certainty about what may have caused the respiratory phobia, or, for that matter, even if Teddy really has one. It's just an hypothesis, probably just one of several that could explain why he talks in that odd way. I've tried to think of other explanations, because there are dangers in believing your first hunch, but I can't come up with any. Also, I've tried to find evidence that would enable me to reject the guess that Teddy has such a phobia. But he does sleep with his arms outside the covers, and he does dislike to suck his milk through a straw and he does lick that sucker rather than suck it, and he is afraid to go swimming and he has had asthmatic attacks and night terrors."

I filled my pipe and continued. "But let me make a confession that will show that I'm far from being any Sherlock Holmes. I once worked with a little girl who had articulation errors somewhat similar to Teddy's, though her speech was much more intelligible. She also showed the other behaviors such as fearing to suck through a straw and sleeping with her arms above the covers, and almost every night she too had terrible nightmares. Once she even told me, "If I close my mouth, I will die!" Because of polio, this girl had spent three months in an iron lung and several more months wearing a chest respirator, so she had good reason for her concern. Anyway, when she was convinced that she could always inhale through her nose even though her mouth was closed, her misarticulations disappeared almost magically."

My colleague was still dubious. "Well, as you say, your hypothesis seems pretty far-fetched," she remarked, "but just suppose it is valid. Then what do I do with Teddy?"

A program was outlined. Use some classical conditioning procedures to get Teddy to tolerate closing off the oral airway, first with his hand and then with his lips and tongue for longer and longer periods, first in silence, then with silent exhalations through the nose and then with vocalization. Do a lot of inhalation-exhalation through the nose. Using hierarchies, get him to combine words together in larger strings, first speaking them on inhalation, then on exhalation after they have been practiced correctly singly. Use a lot of positive suggestion and get him to read, think and say to himself such sentences as "I can always breathe through my nose." Teach him to be a ventriloquist of sorts, manipulating a dummy's or a puppet's mouth and using a hypernasal voice. Have him do most of his inhalation for speech through his nose. Use your operant techniques to get him to hold an object such as a candy cane with his lips closed firmly about it. Get him to prolong the /m/ and /n/ sounds for longer and longer durations. Cumulatively increase the number of syllables spoken on one exhalation. Use humor and food and relaxation as counter-conditioners. Oh, I forget just what I told her but most of it was in this vein. She said she'd give it a try.

I did not see my friend from the public schools again for some time, but I did get a tape from her in the mail. When I played the cassette, it was Teddy talking and he was talking very well. First he read a passage containing all the speech sounds and I heard only one error, the substitution of an /f/ for a /p/ in a blend. Then he spoke spontaneously of some of the fun things he had been doing in speech and it was completely intelligible, though there were a few more errors than when he had read. But it ended with one very clear, perfect sentence, spoken very carefully, and evidently thoroughly rehearsed: "Not so elementary, Sherlock Holmes."

I have presented this diagnostic account not at all to demonstrate my own cleverness, but to demonstrate clearly the necessity for studying our clients thoroughly and for devising hypotheses that will account for their deviant speech behaviors. There is a *why* behind every *what*. Far too often I have been unable to find its answer but always the question must be asked.

Diagnosis, of course, does not stop with the initial examination. As therapy proceeds, the answers to the questions *What?* and *Why?* often change because the client changes, and so does the clinical relationship. New problems, new questions arise continually. Student clinicians often forget this. After the original diagnostic examination has led to a therapy plan and the objectives have been stated, beginning clinicians too often follow that plan slavishly and then they wonder why they fail.

Diagnosis: A Continuing Process

In cleaning out some of my voluminous files, many folders of clinical notes were discarded, for I have always made a practice of jotting down what seemed to have occurred during a therapy session and then reviewing the material often. It's so easy to forget what proved successful or what failed. It's so difficult to demand accountability of oneself, to admit error, even sometimes to recognize progress. Most of these clinical notes consisted of brief statements and questions, but I found one folder dating back to the 1940's which was more detailed. Although I would hate to have them viewed as a model, these notes do seem to illustrate something of what goes on inside the clinician's head as he works with a client. It shows that *diagnosis is a continuing process*.

Bill P. 22 yrs. H.S. education. Employed in an office of a local paperbox factory. Self referred. Boss wants to promote him but says he sounds too drunk to do the intensive phone work involved. Has severe lateral lisp with salivary bubble in emission sometimes. About to get married. Strong motivation??? Seems OK. Should have enough.

SESSION 1. Examination today: Articulation testing: No other errors except lateral emission on /s/ and /z/ and /tS/ and /dʒ/ in all positions in all words. Lateral lisp completely consistent. Found no key words or nonsense combinations that had a single good sibilant. Bill makes the *s* and *z* sounds with a half inch dental gap. Teeth OK though. No jaw thrust nor tongue protrusion. Puts tongue tip against alveolar ridge, and airflow comes around right side of tongue on all sibilants and affricates. (Found this out by tapping cheeks as Bill prolonged the sounds.) No air flow differences between *s* and *z*. Slushy sound, quite noticeable. Does sound almost drunk at times. No error differences when rate, loudness or phonetic contexts are varied except worse in combinations with adjacent sibilants. Easy to see why. Must be some key word or key combination somewhere. What one? Try to get it after final *f* and *v* as in *chiefs* or *calves*. Doesn't recognize his errors at all. Vaguely knows only that he doesn't talk right. How to make him aware? How to stop airflow around right side of tongue?

SESSION 2.   Discrimination practice. Had him prolong his defective *s* and *z* into cupped hand leading to right ear while I inserted the standard *s* and *z* sounds into his left ear along with samples of his own lateral lisp. Used pulses of sound. Bill finally got so he could tell when I put in my imitations of his error and when I made standard sounds. Good technique. What ratio would be best? Suggestion: have him prolong his error sounds as I gradually make my stimulus sound first softly, then louder and louder until he can tell if I'm making his error sound or the standard. Too complicated? But he's got to recognize his error and the difference. How big must a difference be to be a difference perceptually? To be or not to be!

SESSION 3.   Started discrimination training again. Bill more successful but getting bored with tasks. Wants to make the sounds correctly right now. Impatient bugger. Outlined entire course of therapy: need for recognition of characteristics of error; stimulation; learning to make the good sounds; strengthening them; putting them into all his speech gradually; being able to alternate the right and wrong sounds under speed and stress, etc. He responded well to this map. Should have done it earlier. I modeled entire sequence. Should do this with all clients. Had him tap my cheek as I made a correct *s* and then to tap his own when he made defective one. Good response. Showed him his dental gap between upper and lower teeth in a mirror as compared to mine on the sibilants. He tried to do what I did but clenched his teeth too hard and still got defective emission. Time ran out and we ended on failure. Ach!

SESSION 4.   Began again with discrimination. Had him identify errors and correct sounds in isolation, words and connected speech, then listen to his own productions in similar material and watch dental opening in mirror and palpate cheek during sibilant production. Getting better at it but is restless. Got to move faster but hate to do so while discrimination errors still continue. Bill asked repeatedly to be shown how to do it right. Told him he had to hear it first. Mistake? Did a little exploration trying to get correct /s/ from strong visual and auditory stimulation. Failed. Must find other way. Came close to getting one by using *fs* (laughs) and *vz* (calves) on theory that assimilation might bring teeth together. Also it seems harder for him to shift from *f* to *sh* than from *f* to *s*. Got to get him to occlude teeth and stop anchoring tongue on alveolar ridge. Airflow must go down midline and off tip, not around base of upthrust tongue. Damn!

Had Bill use oral inhalation and exhalation, gradually closing teeth on the latter. Then had him suck air in through closed teeth, then repeat as I compressed right cheek to make an /s/ on inhalation. Better! Still mushy and bubbly but I did hear a few bits of high frequency sibilant sounds. Why? The dental frication I suppose. Both of us were tired at end of session and he was discouraged. Hope I don't lose him before I find the answer.

SESSION 5.   Knowing we had to get that tongue tip down, I demonstrated the low-tongued /s/, anchoring the tip at the base of the lower teeth, then closing my teeth, and sucking air in, then blowing it out to produce a good standard /s/. Had him imitate me at every step and gave him strong stimulation at the final one. Glory be! Got a perfect /s/. And he knew it too. Compared it with his usual lateral emission *s* and he heard and felt the difference. Practiced it a few times slowly and weakly. Told him it was weak and fragile and not to try to use it in his speech yet.

According to my notes, this was the crucial therapy session. The newly acquired standard sound was strengthened, incorporated into all kinds of communication, and in another month his lateral lisp was gone. Diagnosis is a continuing process.

THERAPY

"I'm scared," the young clinician said, "I'm petrified. Today I have my first therapy session with my first client and I don't know if I can go through with it. I'm all mixed up and panicky. I've been waiting for this day for a long time, but now I don't know if I am really fitted to be a speech pathologist or not. All those courses in phonetics and speech science, anatomy and linguistics and introduction to speech pathology are behind me but I don't know what to do. I feel inadequate, incompetent. I'm not ready to do my practicum and I don't think I'll ever be. I'm thinking of quitting."

The First Client

I forget what I told her, but I'm sure that I probably said that most beginning clinicians had the same feelings of ambivalence and anxiety when they first recognized the awesome responsibility for shaping another person's life, and that I, who had worked with speech handicapped individuals for so many years, still felt inadequate whenever a new client was confronted for the first time. Human beings are so complex; their equations are always full of unknowns. Each new client is unique; each one comes to us with a history we can never know fully; and each one is being influenced by many forces over which we have no control. Any clinician who feels absolutely confident or competent at such a time is probably insensitive, egocentric or stupid.

I also probably told her that most of her anxiety would fade as soon as she started to think about her client's needs and feelings rather than her own, and that when she did, she would know what to do or at least know how to begin. And I probably expressed some of the basic philosophy that has guided many others: you can only give what you have to give but you have to give all of it. You have to sign the invisible contract stating that you will do your damndest to help that client. I know I would have emphasized the word "help," for that is all any of us can do. No clinician ever cured a client. We contrive conditions and provide experiences so that his speech and language behaviors—and he himself—will change, but the client is the one who does the changing. I'm sure I would also have told that student that, if she signed that contract, she would find many ways to help her client heal his hurt. I also would have insisted that all of us make mistakes, few of which matter in the long run, and that she would probably be surprised (as I have often been) by how much she could really do. And then I probably thought of my own first client.

Cherie was her name. Her case history folder, a thin one, said only that she was the daughter of a very wealthy businessman, an importer, who had committed suicide when Cherie was about ten years old. She had been educated privately by tutors and governesses, then placed in a convent school until she was eighteen, then sent to the university where I was beginning a doctoral program in psychology. Her very severe stuttering had begun suddenly, in fact at exactly 10:32 A.M. on Friday, January 16th of her junior year, a few weeks after her twenty-first birthday. She was halfway through the reading of a poem before a class in Oral Interpretation when it happened. Suddenly she had found herself repeating a syllable interminably, then being completely blocked and mute, then being able to utter a few more words, only to block again. Cherie was immediately referred to the newly established speech clinic, but after two months of group and individual therapy, she not only had not improved but had become much worse.

I've always suspected that the head of that clinic assigned Cherie to me in order to dissuade me from entering the new field of speech pathology. He had refused to allow me to enroll in the few undergraduate courses that were then being offered because I already had my master's degree. (In Old English and Physics!) He also said that I was far too sensitive, poetic and vulnerable to be a good therapist. "You aren't tough enough!" he insisted. "Even though you have overcome your own stuttering fairly well, I don't think stutterers should ever become speech therapists. Go into research or do mental testing or write magazine articles or chop wood for a living. You are just not the kind of a person we need in this field."

But I was not to be discouraged so easily. Barred from the classes in speech correction, I enrolled myself as a candidate for the doctoral degree in psychology and took as many courses as were available in that field. I read the handful of books that dealt with speech disorders. Spending a lot of time in the speech clinic as an observer, I also covertly helped some of the stutterers to do their outside speech assignments, and generally made myself useful. I was determined to help others to share my own wonderful experience of throwing off the shackles of abnormality, of finally gaining the human birthright, the ability to speak. I knew there were no jobs in speech pathology, but perhaps as a clinical psychologist I could specialize and create my own clinic for stutterers someday.

So it was a surprise when one day the director called me in and told me I could have Cherie as a client. I must say that I didn't trust the grin that flickered under his mustache, for, of all the stutterers in the clinic, she was the one who probably had the worse prognosis. A spoiled brat, neurotic as hell, a saboteur! Though physically attractive, none of the stutterers or student clinicians liked her, nor did I. "I'm giving you this case because Cherie is a hysterical stutterer and you're the only one around here with some background. (I had undergone psychoanalysis.) Get her out of my hair! Combine speech therapy with psychotherapy. I don't think you can help her but she's all yours." He grinned again sadistically.

I'll never forget how completely inadequate I felt that next morning when I ushered Cherie into a corner of an empty classroom for our first session. What to do? How to begin? She wasn't a bit helpful or cooperative either. At first openly hostile, she challenged me immediately. "What makes you think you can help me?" she demanded, stuttering grotesquely and severely on every word and watching me closely to see if I could bear it without flinching. Many stutterers, consciously or unconsciously, do this testing. They want to be very sure that the person into whose hands they are about to place themselves will not discard them in revulsion. I passed the test easily, not just because I had also been a severe stutterer, but because I was interested in analyzing her stuttering behaviors objectively. Answering Cherie's question was more difficult. I told her bluntly that I wanted to try to help her because she had not progressed at all during the months that she had spent in the clinic, that it was obvious that she was desperately alone and that she needed a guide who knew the wilderness in which she was lost. I told her that I would do my utmost to help her solve her *many* problems. When the word *many* was emphasized, her eyes widened and I detected an almost imperceptible nod. Then I outlined how we would proceed. She would be seen every day for two hours, the first being spent in learning to control her stuttering, and the second in exploring the emotional conflicts that might have caused or were still maintaining it. I was very stern, very professional and I really thought I had been very effective in defining my role in the therapeutic relationship when suddenly Cherie lifted her skirt and with complete fluency asked, "Don't you think I have nice legs?"

I don't remember what I replied. Probably half stammered something about being more interested in her mouth and what was above rather than below it—but I know I ended that first session hurriedly. A shambles! Maybe I should go back to the forest and be that lumberjack. No, damn her, I'd help her if it killed me. She'd won the first round but there would be others.

That was the first skirmish of a battle—no, a war—that continued for several months. I've worked with a horde of stutterers since but never with one so belligerently resistant as Cherie. Every session provoked emotional storms. She would refuse to do what I asked. She would weep copiously, curse me, plaster me with venom. Once she even slapped my face and when she did, I grabbed her arms and told her that if she did it again I'd knock her teeth in, and then I would pick her up and we'd continue our therapy as though nothing had happened. Sometimes she would refuse to talk at all, glowering with hatred for as long as half an hour. When she did this, I waited calmly, watching her. There also were several instances when Cherie even ran out of the room, but she always returned. It was a traumatic introduction to the field of speech pathology.

Each day, the first hour, the speech therapy portion, was the worst. We would sit together before a large mirror and try to keep her stuttering from becoming involuntary, to maintain control of that jerking jaw, to hunt for phonation when there was none, to smooth out her tremors, to decrease the tension. When she stuttered, I stuttered right with her and in the same way, but very calmly. I showed her how unnecessary her struggle was, and modeled a better way of releasing. I rewarded her for feeling the fluency she did have. I helped her to recognize the abnormal postures that triggered her blocks and showed her how to change them. Cherie fought me every inch of the way, tooth and nail, fang and claw, as I dragged her screamingly from the morass of self-defeating behaviors in which she had immersed herself.

Our second hour was usually not so traumatic. I did not play psychiatrist, but rather listened day after day to the torrent of emotion that accompanied the telling of her life story in the utmost, but often superficial, detail. An only child. An unwanted child. A cold mother who viewed her as an encumbrance to her life in high society. An aloof father who while he lived had lavished her with expensive toys and gifts but whom she rarely saw. He had killed himself and she had heard the shot and found the body. Cherie didn't want to talk about it. The parents had travelled constantly, leaving Cherie in the hands of a succession of governesses, only one of whom had shown the girl a few crumbs of affection. She told of a cook who had befriended her and been discharged because she had forgotten "her place," and of a gardener who occasionally had been kind. Cherie had never had any real playmates.

The world Cherie pictured for me was as strange as a moonscape. I tried hard to understand and to show her when I did, and when I did not. The hardest part was to try to separate her facts from her fantasies, for she lied to me a lot, and sometimes just to boobytrap me. For example, when she told repeatedly of her life in the convent school, a very strict one, the versions varied widely from session to session. Once, after a blatantly fraudulent account about a nun who had whipped her, Cherie stopped suddenly and asked me if I believed her. I said no, but that I was more interested in the emotion she was expressing than in whether the whipping had actually occurred, and I was wondering if she was really telling me how she felt about her own mother's rejection. Whoops! Mount Cherie erupted again, covering me with the volcanic ash of her stuttering and hatred. So it went, day after day.

Beginning clinicians are always troubled by self-doubts, thinking that only they have such thoughts of inadequacy. I certainly felt that way. Now I know that even the very best therapists share that experience over and over again. Indeed, it is salutory in that it helps us to recognize our limitations. Sometimes it even leads to personal growth, since our mistakes and failures, when honestly confronted, have in them the seeds of change. One can fall backward or forward; one can *fail* forward too.

But I didn't know that when I was Cherie's clinician. There were so many mistakes made that I wriggle embarrassingly even now when they come to mind. One of them, though, was almost fatal and I use the word in its literal sense. Cherie had three major stuttering patterns. The first consisted of compulsive runaway repetitions of a syllable or word. This was our first target of therapy and in a few months it was eliminated. The second pattern consisted of a silent lip protrusion accompanied by tremor. This too was readily modified once she could confront it, fake it, and vary it enough to get control. But the third pattern caused us much more difficulty. Cherie would spasmodically jerk her jaw downward so that her mouth was widely agape and then she would be unable to utter any sound at all. As she froze in this position, her eyes would glaze and then her eyelids would cover them. She looked so much like a person with the *petit mal* kind of epilepsy that I had her checked at the university hospital, but the report was entirely negative. (They did provide the important information that Cherie stuttered.)

But to return to the mistake that was almost fatal: one day we had been working hard on this third kind of stuttering behavior while Cherie was making phone calls. She had failed over and over again to modify it and was weeping when I took her hands and placed them on her mouth and jaws so that she could have some contact with the self when she was in the throes of her blocking. That failed too, but suddenly she took my hands in hers and had them stroke her face and, lo! The phonation came instantly. We were both astonished. Cherie made another phone call and again the same thing happened. Repeatedly, all I had to do was to stroke or pat her face and the hard blocking terminated immediately. "To hell with this," I exclaimed. "No more laying on of hands! No tricks, you damned neurotic woman!" She wept but I was adamant. I was a scientist, not a shaman. I would not do any faith healing. Looking back from the vantage of years of therapy, I am appalled. She was trying to tell me something and I would not listen. I was not sensitive to Cherie's needs; I was thinking only of my own.

The following day, everything went badly and it was a relief when the session ended. It was a very cold, nasty day outside with sleet and slush.

Cherie offered me a ride to my room a mile away, as she had often done before, but this time I accepted. I knew I shouldn't have said yes, but it was a long walk, I had a bad cold, and so on. Well, we got into her Cadillac coupe and she drove like a maniac across town. I tried to get her to slow down. I tried to give her directions. I told her to stop and let me out! She didn't seem to hear me! Then she started to say something just as we came to a main street where a trolley car was coming right toward us, clanging its bell furiously. I yelled at Cherie and pointed but she was in one of those long hard blocks we had been working on, mouth open, eyes glazed. Worst of all, as I hunched down to wait for the inevitable crash, I saw her eyelids begin to close tightly. When the trolley car missed us by inches, I grabbed the keys out of the ignition, stopped the car and left her there in the middle of the street, still blocking, still trying to tell me something. To hell with speech pathology! To hell with Cherie! I went to my room and drank half a pint of whiskey before I could gain any sort of calm. Phew!

You can be sure that in the sessions that followed I worked very hard to show Cherie how to release herself from the hard stuttering that had almost killed us, but to no avail. Referring once to the incident, she said, "But why didn't you touch me? Why didn't you release me?" Again, I did not hear her message.

I devoted several psychotherapy sessions in vainly exploring the onset of Cherie's stuttering. What was the poem she had been reading to the class when the stuttering first occurred? She could not remember it. We repeatedly re-enacted the scene with Cherie on the stage and me as the audience. I asked her to make up a poem, any poem, or to recite the first one that came into her head. First she recited Vachel Lindsay's "The Leaden Eyed," beginning with: "Let not young souls be smothered out/ before they do quaint deeds and fully flaunt their pride." She said she had forgotten the rest. Then, after a long silence, Cherie began to cry again and through her sobs I heard, "Breath and death! Breath and death! And who but I could hear that cry?" I had her repeat it over and over again until it lost all meaning. I even asked her to do some free association on the key words, but nothing came. Woefully amateurish psychotherapy it was, and completely ineffective. I was just too incompetent and I knew it.

Several weeks later in one of our psychotherapy sessions, Cherie recounted a dream. She was in a rowboat without oars being carried down a roaring river toward a great falls. I was on the bank smoking my pipe and didn't hear her call for help. She said that she had had other similar dreams. "What did they mean?" she asked. Instead of replying, I asked her to tell me. She could not.

By this time, we had achieved a pretty good relationship. Cherie no longer battled me so furiously. Often she tried to do the things I asked. She brought me crazy little gifts which I dumped into the nearest wastebasket. She shyly told me that she liked and trusted me and hoped that I liked her. I told her brusquely that I didn't need her liking—that I was there to help her solve her problem, period, paragraph, not very truly yours—and now let's get to work. I was fearful of transference, I know now, afraid to use that powerful but dangerous tool. I was her therapist. She was my client and that was all.

Shortly after the trolley incident, the tempo of therapy accelerated. Except for an occasional hard blocking of the kind she had in the car with me, most of her speech became fairly fluent. In our psychotherapy sessions she was able to verbalize much deeper material than ever before and to do so more honestly. Only two topics did she seem to avoid—death and sex—though she did tell me again about finding her father's body after he had killed himself. She narrated that scene with a curious lack of emotion, as though it was something she had observed in a movie. As for her love life, she continually gave me the impression that it was nil, until one day she told me this incredible tale.

Cherie began by asking if I were a virgin and so, of course, I replied by asking why she had asked the question. "Well, I am," she responded, "But I've also been married." I could not conceal my surprise. "Yes, I ran away and got married to the first boy who showed any interest in me. He was a poor student who waited on tables in our dormitory. I don't really think Tommy really wanted to get married at all, but I told him I had an income of my own and we'd go through college together on my money. You know how impetuous I am. Coming out of that convent school and free for the first time in my life, I was desperate for a close relationship, the closer the better. No, I didn't tell my mother, which was just as well because I had to have the marriage annulled. Anyway, I dragged poor Tommy to the justice of the peace for the ceremony, which was horrid, and then drove him to the cottage I had rented at a nearby lake for our weekend honeymoon." Cherie wept for a long time before continuing.

"Well, after a good dinner and a long walk on the beach, we came back to the cottage. When Tommy took off his clothes and got into bed, I was filled with panic. Just terrified! I couldn't do it! I couldn't! Oddly enough, I remember recalling what an old governess of mine had said about being sure to open the bedroom window on my wedding night so the bluebird could fly in. I knew better, of course, having spent four years in that convent school, but at that moment, I . . . I just couldn't bear losing . . . my . . . my childhood, so I started to cry wretchedly there in the corner of that room. When I tried to explain, Tommy comforted me, saying that he understood, that he'd be patient with his child bride, that I'd get used to the idea. A nice man. A gentle man. And, bless his heart, he even went along with a crazy idea of mine—that we'd pretend to be children together, and play leap-frog over each other, then jump into bed and go to sleep."

With great difficulty I managed to keep a straight face. "Listen to her!" I commanded myself. "Try to understand. But don't let her fool you again, dammit!" "And then what happened?" I asked. "Did you finally have intercourse?" "No," she almost shouted. "Tommy was so nice, so considerate. He just kissed me, moved to his side of the bed, and finally went to sleep. And snored. I didn't sleep a wink though. Just lay there and shook all night."

"And then?"

"Well, that's the way it went for two more nights. I'd squat down and Tommy would jump over me; then he'd hunch down, and I'd leap over him, and finally into bed. Just like two innocent little children playing on the sand. But the fourth night Tommy would have no more of it. He'd been sort of surly all day, and when we put on our night things, he suddenly banged his fist on the headboard and yelled at me, "No more goddamned leap-frog!""

There was more to the tale but I couldn't hear what Cherie was saying, I was laughing so hard. Outrageous belly laughter that I couldn't control. Just a very dirty, male, chauvinist pig! Dimly, I knew how terribly offended she was, but all I could think of was that poor guy beating on the bed and hollering "No more goddamned leap-frog!" Finally I fled from the room and the wreckage of our relationship.

I must admit there was some relief when Cherie did not show up for her Friday appointment, for I really didn't see how I could face her. I was full of guilt. I berated myself. I had betrayed her. What a lousy therapist I had turned out to be! How could I make amends? What could I say in apology? Could we ever regain the close, trusting relationship we had finally achieved? These questions kept circling in my head along with the impossible, outrageous, intolerable answer: learn to play leap-frog. But I was also very full of anxiety, an anxiety that suddenly flared to gigantic proportions when, that weekend, a florist delivered a box to my door that contained a single red rose and a note that said, "When you read this, I shall be dead. Cherie."

Frantically, I called her dormitory. They told me she had withdrawn from the university and had gone home. I called the director of the clinic and explained what had happened. He just laughed at my tale and my anxiety. "Don't worry. She'll be back to haunt you Monday." I was not so sure. It was a bad time!

But she returned. Cherie had come to say goodbye. No, she wasn't going to kill herself. She had tried—even had the poison bottle to her mouth—but she couldn't do it. But she'd never be afraid again that she would commit suicide like her father had done. She was going away to make a new life for herself. She would get married and have children and give them all the love and caring she had never known. She thanked me for all the help I had given her but she didn't need me any more. My laughter had set her free from me, she said, and she thanked me for that too. She would write me. Before leaving, Cherie took my hands and stroked her face lightly with them. "I have stopped stuttering," she said. "Goodbye." Only then did I realize that she had been completely fluent throughout that long farewell.

I heard from Cherie every Christmas for many years. The notes were very short but always included her thanks for my help. She had married and had children and was happy. And she hadn't ever stuttered again. I still don't know why. Perhaps you do.

Motivation Problems

Perhaps the most important of all the clinical skills required for effective therapy is the clinician's ability to motivate his clients. Most of my own failures, I feel, have occurred because I was unable to do this. Beginning clinicians are shocked when they find that many of their clients resist their efforts to help them. They feel that it isn't fair to find their clients putting forth only a token effort, appearing bored and uninterested or even actively sabotaging. They call them lazy, but personally I have never known a truly lazy client. When I felt like dubbing one with that label, it always turned out that he had different needs and different goals than mine.

Besides, there is always the cost-payoff ratio. There are costs of time, effort, and unpleasantness that must be paid by the client if he is to overcome a speech handicap. The field of speech pathology is no rose garden. Learning and unlearning take time, and often the client (as well as the clinician) thinks, "How long, oh Lord, how long?" The final goal of relief seems so far away in time that the client cannot see it or smell it. For example, most stutterers come to us with unrealistic expectations. They want the magical, miracle cure in a hurry; they want to buy the canary bird for a nickel and are disappointed when they find that learning and unlearning require hard work. Finally, many of the things our clients must experience can be unpleasant. Confronting the fears and flaws of deviancy can give rise to a lot of negative emotion, as can the temporary failures that usually mark the route that must be followed.

The experienced clinician is not personally affronted when he finds a client loafing on the therapeutic job or resisting his remedial program. What he does is to find ways of increasing the client's expectation of pay-off, or ways of decreasing the costs. To do so, he must study his client and know his needs, and he must redesign his program to make the rewards more evident. When the expected cost-payoff ratio is small enough, the needed motivation will be there.

One of the most powerful drives that our clients possess is the need to escape punishment or unpleasantness. When this can be mobilized, it can be a very powerful motivator. I have a story to illustrate this. It is a verbatim transcript of a tape recording made for me by a wonderful old lady when she was eighty-five years old. It recounts very vividly some of the feelings of a child in the last part of the last century who evidently had a mild articulatory problem. It also reflects the belief of that time that a speech defect was a nasty habit to be broken by punishment. I'd like to share it with you, if only to demonstrate that speech pathology has come a long way.

Before I even started school, I had my first very dreadful speaking experience. It happened like this: one summer day I missed my dinner because my mother sent me to the store with my little red wagon and a jar to get some vinegar. At that time we lived on a farm on the outskirts of a small village. My father was a co-owner of the store and the other owner was my uncle, a nice fat jolly man who liked children very much. He was always very kind to me. He would always give me a piece of candy or something of that sort... Anyway, I went to the store and he asked me what I wanted. I told him I wanted some "winegar" because I couldn't say my *v* sounds. My uncle thought that was very funny so he made me say it again, so I did. I kept trying to tell him what I wanted, saying the word vinegar wrong over and over again and over and over again. He laughed. Finally he gave me the vinegar and I took it home. Unfortunately, my father had to go to the store to get some nails, so my uncle told him about my saying "winegar" for vinegar. Only I didn't really say it like that, it was much worse than that. It was very mutilated and distorted, as I recall, and so my father was very angry about it. My father demanded perfection not only in himself but in all of us. He came home just storming and so we knew something was up when he came in the door. He called me outside and I knew I must have done something wrong, though I didn't know what it was. Father took a whip. He had a very big buggy whip and sometimes if the offenses were minor he would switch us with the willow switch, and if the offenses were very big he would use the buggy whip. This time he started with the willow switch so I figured it wasn't going to be too bad, that maybe it would hurt, but I could cry it out and then it would be all over anyway in a few hours.

But my father looked at me hard and said, "Say vinegar!" So I said "winegar," or whatever it was, and he switched me and I cried of course. He kept demanding that I say it right and kept telling me to repeat it after him, but I kept repeating it wrong. He was even yelling it at me, but I couldn't say it right. This infuriated Father so much that he got the big buggy whip and he spanked me very hard with it. I even bled in a few places. It was a very brutal and cruel whipping. Finally he gave up and he said, "You'll learn to say that word by tomorrow morning or you'll get another whipping." Then I was sent to my room upstairs, my bedroom, and was given a glass of water and a piece of crusted bread which was standard punishment after anything like that. I had to stay there for all that day. The thing that saved me (I don't know what would have happened if it hadn't) was my older sister, ten years older, who had come back from boarding school. She had always given me a great deal of attention and I loved her deeply. When I was born she liked me because I was so tiny. She thought I was a little doll and so she always protected me and took care of me, and had this motherly feeling toward me. Anyway she said, "Honey, I'll tell you how to say it. Say 'vinegar.'" And I said "winegar" or whatever it was. She said, "No, that's wrong," and she thought and thought and walked around the room awhile. Pretty soon she came back and she said, "You know Vin (Vincent) Mitchell?" I said, "Yes," and she said, "Well, say Vin Mitchell's name." So I did, I said, "Vin." "That's part of vinegar, vin-vinegar," my sister told me. Now say "VIN again," so I said "VIN," and then she took a block, an alphabet block, and said, "What's this letter?" and I said "E" and she said, "Well, now you say 'E.' First say Vin Mitchell's name and say 'E,' and I said Vin Mitchell E." My sister laughed, "Vin . . . E." Then my sister said, "Do you remember old Garfield Smith?" "Yes," I replied, "old Garfield Smith, I remember him. He fought in the civil war." Then my sister said, "Now you say his name, and put it with Vin and E." So I thought about it and I said, "Vin . . . E . . . Garfield Smith." "No," said my sister, "you say, Vin . . . e . . . and then say only Gar, only the first part of his name: GAR."

Well that's how I learned to say "Vin . . . e . . . gar. Vin . . . E . . . gar." I said it a million times, all day and all night so I could say it to my father in the morning. I woke up very early in the morning, and of course I was feeling very painful all over, but my mother put some bear grease on my body so it felt some better, physically anyway, and she comforted me, and my sister was comforting me too. Anyway, next morning I went before my father and I was crying and sobbing but I managed to get out "VIN . . . E . . . GAR," "VIN . . . E . . . GAR" just like that. Well, he thought he'd won the battle and that I had learned my lesson. If so, I learned the hard way. It's so hard for a little child to talk right.

The old lady shed a tear or two, then continued. Here's another similar experience. When I was a very small child in school somewhere about the second or third grade, I had another dreadful experience of the same sort. I was expelled from school for saying "mosquito" wrong. We had teachers then who had only gone through high school and they really didn't know very much about teaching. Yes, that was a long time ago. Anyway, this teacher (I think she was only nineteen and she was out teaching all the children of rural schools, some of whom were older than she was) was having a spelling lesson and we had the word "mosquito." Well, I called it "moskweeto." "Say 'mosquito,'" she demanded. So once again I said "moskweeto." Well, we went on that way all day long—every once in a while she'd try me with "mosquito" and I'd say it wrong, always thinking I was saying it right. Finally, she accused me of being sassy and impudent and she said, "Say it right!" I said, "I am saying it right." Finally she said, "You go home! I'm going to expel you and you can't come back to school until you say it right."

It was really very dreadful and I was so emotionally upset I wanted to die. I was . . . I just . . . was just a very little girl. I felt life was not worth living unless I could say mosquito and that something evil was possessing me. It was a very dreadful emotional ordeal, especially when my father heard about it. He told me to say "mosquito" right and go back to school the next morning and apologize to the teacher. He was director of the school, he said, and he wasn't going to have his child get into any trouble with the teacher and so forth. I must mind the teacher or else! I remembered the buggy whip. I didn't know what to do. Once again my sister was my savior. By chance she was invited to a party and so she came home on Thursday night I guess, or Wednesday . . . or somewhere around the middle of the week, anyway, and so, when she found out what had happened, she came up to my room where I was once again on bread and water, "I'll tell you how to say it. You say Eenie-Meenie-Minie-Mo." Well, we had played that game a lot, so I said, "Eenie-Meenie-Minie-Mo." "Now you say 'mo,'" she suggested and so I said, "Mo." "Well, that was all right," she commented.

Then after she thought a while, she went outside and was gone a long, long time and while she was away I said the word over and over, "Mo-Mo." Finally she came back and she had gone to the cupboard where the winter things were kept and got a pair of skis. She brought out a ski and she said, "Now, do you know how to say ski?" "Of course," I said. "Ski." Then she said, "Now you say 'MO' and then ski." So I said, "Mosqui . . ." and then she said, "What's that down there inside your stocking? Take your shoe off." So I took my shoe off and she said, "What's THAT?" I said, "That's my toe." "Well now, say Mo-ski-toe." So I said "mosquito" just the way it should be said and I kept saying it for hours, until morning came. I said "mosquito" to my father and I managed to get back to the school on Friday morning, but I had to apologize to the teacher before all the children who laughed at me even though I could say it right. That hurt me worse than anything else. It's awful to be ridiculed by your friends and classmates. Then the teacher gave all of us a great talk about behaving and she ridiculed me also. It was hard being a little girl who couldn't talk right. I sort of hate to tell all this about myself, but if it might help some child to be helped with her speech then it is worthwhile.

My second tale might be entitled "The Latrine Treatment of Stuttering." It concerns a client whom I could not motivate to do anything at all, and yet who became very fluent when the United States Army took charge.

This happened during World War II, when there was a very large army camp about twenty miles from Kalamazoo at Battle Creek. One morning, two officers and a private came to my office. "Sir," said the older officer, "we need your help. I'll come to the point immediately. Yesterday we had a review and inspection by the general commanding this entire area. It was going very well and we were proud of our men when the general suddenly accosted this soldier (he pointed to the private) and said, 'Son, what's your name and number?' Well, in answering him, this man spit in the general's face. You see, he spits when he stutters. Well, the front ranks laughed and the laughter spread all over the parade ground. All our training and preparations were shattered. Well, sir, the general apologized to soldier Murphy here and said in effect that I should see that this man was cured pronto or he'd have the scalp of every officer in the battalion. And that he'd be back in two months to make sure. Sir, the United States Army needs you.'' (I almost saluted) ''You can have him day or night,'' he continued, ''and you can have any resource or aid we can provide. Will you cure him? I insist, sir, that you must.''

Murphy was the ''laziest'' client I have ever had. He never participated in the group sessions; just ogled the girl clinicians or dozed. All of his outside speech tasks were done in the local bars and performed perfunctorily if they were done at all. My own individual therapy sessions with him went no better. I learned to duck when he stuttered and sprayed everything in sight with saliva, but Sleepy Murphy learned nothing at all. Finally, fed up with his resistance, I told him to start working or get the hell out. ''Aw now Doc,'' he protested, ''you don't understand (I had to watch out for those *st* words or I'd have to wipe my face). I been in this man's army for three years and I never had it so good. Got my own jeep now, and a driver. No drill. I sleep late when the other guys are out on the range or doing push-ups. I tell 'em I gotta get my sleep and relax. I get steak when they get beans—protein, you know. I got it made, Doc. All these good-looking girls to talk to in the Tallyho or fool around with. I get cured of my goddam stuttering and I'm back there doggin' it with the rest of the grunts. No way, Doc. No way!'' I grinned, but told him I'd give him another week to shape up or ship out.

But I did not have to dismiss him. That very afternoon when he was careening around the city with his jeep full of girls, all half-tight, he had a collision with the car driven by our mayor's wife. Sleepy was taken to jail. The next Monday morning as I entered my office, I was confronted by the older officer who had brought Sleepy to us. He didn't salute but again came right to the point. ''Sir,'' he said, ''you have failed the United States Army.'' When I tried to explain by citing Murphy's lack of effort and cooperation, a gleam came to his eyes. ''You mean you've taught him what to do but he won't do it? Oh ho!'' He clicked his heels as he left and I sighed with some unprofessional and unpatriotic relief. ''Well, that's the last I'll see of Sleepy,'' I thought.

But it wasn't. About six months later I had to give a speech on motivation and learning to a bunch of teachers in the Kellogg Auditorium at Battle Creek and was well under way when suddenly I saw Murphy in the front row, grinning broadly. So I told my audience his tale to illustrate the importance of motivation, and because I was curious, I asked Sleepy to come up to corroborate the point I was making, namely that unless you wanted to learn, you wouldn't. To my surprise, he came up on the platform, and then he told them I was dead wrong, and that he'd learned plenty from me. But what shocked me most was that the man was very fluent. No spitting or spraying, just a few little easy prolongations or repetitions. Not many of them, either, so I asked him what had happened.

No one yet has ever believed me, and I'm not sure I do either, but I swear by my birch tree that this is the tale he told us.

"Well, Doc. It was like this. You know that little major who brung me over to you. Well, when he got me out of jail, he read me the riot act. Blistered me good. And he tells me you said that I knew how to talk OK but wouldn't try. He said he'd what you call it . . . oh, mo-ti-vate me good. So he takes me to the latrine and sez that I'm going live there till I get cured. I thought he wuz kidding, Doc, but he wasn't. They bring me my bedroll and I gotta bunk there, and they bring my meals there and they set a guard to make sure I stay there. Geez, Doc. Day after day it goes on. And the other guys, oh, they give me the business every time they come to the can. You know how it is. A week goes by and the major comes. 'What's yer name, soldier?' he asks, and I get stuck and stutter and spit. 'OK,' he sez, 'I'll see you in a week.' Well I got to thinking I'd be there for the duration and I was getting pretty ripe, the smell and all, so I tries to remember what you'd been teaching those other guys at the clinic. Slow and easy. No need to spit. Keep yer mouth moving. Don't get worked up. Well, Doc, I begin to get better, I did. And I even talked good to the major when he come next time until he tells me to say, 'Peter Piper picked a peck of pickled peppers.' That threw me, and Doc, the major, he spits. 'See you next week, soldier,' he sez. God, how I practiced, Doc. Those *p*'s wuz always tough for me. I betcha I say that Piper one million times. I say it to every guy comes in and when the major he come next time I said it good. Three times I had to say it to him and then he asked me my name and number and a lot of other things, but I was watching myself and they come out good too. So he let me out and here I am and I don't spit no more, no sir. I hear you gonna make a speech here so I come thank you. How about a beer, Doc, after you get through?"

Most of us assume that if a client has a severe problem in communication, he will want to get rid of it. This is not always true; he may feel that he may lose more than he could gain. Again we find here the cost-payoff ratio.

I'm sure that every clinician hates to have a client walk out on him—I certainly do. I always feel that it's my fault, not his, and that somehow I have failed to discern his needs. The following client certainly illustrates this.

Lora was a freshman when she came to us. She didn't want to come. She came only when she was failing one of her college courses because of her deafness and because her counselor insisted on referring her. Since this was in the thirties before audiometers were available, I got out my watch and set of tuning forks, and calibrated the office rug with chalk lines, using my own hearing acuity as the standard. Yes, she was deaf—totally deaf in both ears. (I had plugged first one ear then the other with cotton as I tested her.) I wrote out some questions and was surprised to hear a very good voice and almost perfect articulation when she answered them. The inflections were appropriate; there was no monotone; there were only a few minor articulation errors; her language was excellent. I asked Lora aloud how old she had been when the accident or illness had caused her to lose her hearing, thinking that it must have happened fairly recently. "No," she said, "I've been deaf since birth." I was completely surprised. No congenitally deaf person should have such good speech and language. Also, she seemed to be able to understand me without difficulty. She must be a very good lip reader. I asked her some more questions while putting my pipe in my mouth and lighting it and she understood me easily, a feat that even the best lip reader on earth would find difficult. A malingerer? Psychic deafness? But when I put up a filing folder to hide my face, she "heard" nothing. I left the office for a moment and told a student to wait two minutes, then yell and bang the door. He did so very loudly but she didn't jump or show any sign of awareness.

It took me several sessions before I could make any sense out of the picture and even then it didn't make much. It became evident that Lora could hear perfectly only when she was watching the speaker's mouth or face. Incredible, but that's the way it was. I tested her in a hundred ways but the answer was always the same. She heard with her eyes. Fortunately, she came from Grand Rapids, so I went there to see her mother to get some of the history I couldn't get from Lora. The girl didn't want me to go and when I got there I could understand. An old ramshackle house full of poverty. The mother was not very bright, but she did finally provide some insight. She had not known that Lora was deaf until a great aunt, a teacher, had visited them shortly after the girl's first birthday. It was she who had told them that Lora was deaf and dumb (she had not begun to talk) and that she had to find someone to teach the girl sign language and lip reading right away. A deaf couple who lived down the street away agreed to help. Lora lived at home but went to them for lessons every afternoon, and soon she was talking. Indeed, they were so proud of the girl's lip reading and signing ability that they were now sending her to college so she could become a teacher of the deaf. They told the mother that Lora was the best lip reader in the world. I had to agree.

What to do? Somehow I had to free the girl from her dependence on the visual cues that opened the auditory gates in her nervous system—if that indeed was what was wrong. So I tried having Lora intermittently open and shut her eyes as she listened to the directions I gave her verbally. Very little success. Then I tried putting first one and then several layers of cheese cloth over my face as I talked. She could understand me if I used one layer but not two. One night I worked with her in my darkened office, moving a flashlight further and further and further away from my face. No results. I was about to give up, when one day while I was talking to her, I took my pipe out of my mouth and found that she heard me even when her eyes followed the pipe. Aha! I immediately instituted a training program in which I placed my thumb and forefinger horizontally upon my lips and squeezed them together with every syllable I spoke. Though my lips were pretty well covered she understood me easily. Then very gradually I kept beating out the syllables but asked her to watch my thumb-finger closing as I moved my hand further and further away from my face. She finally could hear what was said even when my arm was outstretched and far from my mouth. Then I faded out the visual pinching stimulus by lessening my thumb and forefinger movements until all she had to do was to look at my fingers in order to comprehend.

What next? I began to lower my hand and finally put it in my pocket and asked her to imagine that it was pinching as I talked. That was the breakthrough, though for some time she had to keep my fingers in her mind's eye when she listened to me. The transfer to other speakers was also difficult at first, but progress moved swiftly from that point and very soon she could hear what people were saying even with her eyes closed. (She just had to imagine they were moving their lips.) We were both exhilarated with her "new ears."

I should have known better—should have had more sense—should have anticipated what might happen. Summer vacation intervened and although we still had more to do, Lora didn't show up when school resumed in the fall. I waited and waited. Finally, I found that she had dropped out of school. I went to Lora's home in Grand Rapids, but she was living with the deaf couple who had befriended her. I finally tracked her down to discover that she had gone back to hearing with her eyes. I could tell she felt sorry for me, but she wasn't coming back. She explained that being a hearing person in a hearing world had been too hard an adjustment, that all of her friends were deaf, that she belonged to the deaf sub-culture, that she considered the deaf couple to be more her true parents than her real ones were, that she didn't know how to get along with hearing people and so on. And besides, trying to listen only with one's ears was too much hard labor. I learned something from Lora. No, I learned a lot!

Here is another anecdote that makes much the same point.

One morning a phone call came in from the Michigan State Police post in a neighboring town. It was from Trooper Pat Brown, a fine man with whom I'd gone rabbit hunting several times. "Doc," he said, "we need your help. This morning we picked up a man who's deaf or dumb or crazy. No, he's not really deaf. Seems to understand what we say OK, and he's not dumb either. He talks, but we can't understand a word of his gibberish. No identification. No driver's license. Went through a stop sign on M-26. Can you come over?" I asked if the man could read or write. No. About how old was he? About thirty. Had he shown any signs of having had a stroke? No. Was he an escapee from our State Hospital for the Insane? No, they'd checked that right away. Were they sure he could understand what they said to him? Yes. I said I'd be over to see him right away.

When I got to the police post I found their information to be correct. The man was almost completely unintelligible. Even using the skills that had enabled me to comprehend utterances of children with delayed speech and language that their own mothers could not understand, I was able to guess the identity of only a few standard words in his excited torrent of jargon. Words such as "I," "no," "tah" (call or car?), "wipe" (wife), and "piddin taytuh" (filling station?) occurred over and over again as he tried to make us understand. All of them were questionable except "I" and "no." I was able to guess his words for "filling station" only because he acted out the process of filling a gas tank. "What's your name?" "Wih-uh-doh." "Wi-uh-doh!" he shouted pointing to himself, "Wi-uh-doh!" The poor devil was almost beside himself with frustration and so were we when the phone rang. It was Mrs. William Jones, the man's wife.

Pat, my trooper friend, talked to her for several minutes and then said she wanted to talk to her husband. What a mess of incoherent utterance! We couldn't understand a single thing he said, but he was obviously speaking in long sentences with familiar inflections and it was apparent that he was communicating easily. Finally he stopped and handed the phone back to Pat. "OK, OK," Pat said to the wife. "We won't book him and we'll bring him home, but for God's sake give us directions. We can't make out anything he says." Hanging up, he asked me if I would drive the man in his truck and follow him in the police car; then he'd bring me back to the post. I agreed.

When I saw the old ramshackle truck I wished I hadn't: a haywire special of ancient vintage. When we got in and I could not follow the man's garbled instructions, he had to get it started, but finally we were rattling on our way through the countryside. And finally we got to his home, a run-down farm house on a little knoll overlooking some old barns and sheds. A few goats watched the three of us parade up to the back door.

To our surprise, the house was very clean and neat and so was his wife. After giving William fits for taking the truck and then listening to his long incoherent (to us) explanation of what had happened, she told us about him. He had never learned to talk right, so he never went to school or learned to read or write. William's mother was born deaf; his father had died early. William had been a hired man on her folks' farm and she had learned his language and learned to like him. Their two kids could understand him perfectly, too. A fine man, she said. A fine, happy man. Easy to live with. Never caused any trouble before. Had never taken the truck to town without her, but she had been pretty sick that morning and they needed the kerosene for the chickencoop heater badly what with its being so cold and three settings of new chicks just starting to run around. And so. . . .

Well, the trooper laid down the law. William wasn't to drive anywhere outside the farm itself. No matter what! He had to have a license and if he couldn't read or write or talk he couldn't get one. Understand? They both nodded. They understood. Pointing to himself, William said several paragraphs of unintelligibility. His wife translated, "He says he knows that's the law and that he won't ever break it again and he thanks you for not putting him in jail and he's sorry he caused you so much trouble bringing him back and all and having such a hard time." At this point William broke in with some more of his jargon. "And he says he wishes he could read and write and talk but he can't. He never had a chance to go to school. . . ."

The trooper was touched. "Damned shame," he said. Then, turning to me, he asked, "Doc, why don't you take this guy on? Give the poor devil a chance to learn to talk anyway. Nobody should have to try to get along like that." Knowing a bit about what the prospect entailed, I hesitated, a reaction Pat took for agreement. He turned to the two of them. "How about it? Doc here is a speech doctor down at the college in Kalamazoo. He can teach you to talk right. And maybe to read and write too. You want to try it?" William looked at me a bit dubiously, but his wife seemed mildly enthusiastic—at least until the little matter of transportation arose. I told them I'd have to see him for an hour at least three times a week for several months—and even then I couldn't guarantee success. It would mean that both of them would have to come three mornings every week. Travel time would be an hour each way. Could they spare that time? And would that old truck hold up? Pat brushed aside the latter objection. "Hell, Doc, if it breaks down, I'll get the guys down at the police garage to fix it. OK, you two be down at the speech clinic tomorrow morning," he commanded. "At what time, Doc? Ten o'clock? OK You be there, understand?" They nodded and I told the wife how to find our speech clinic. Lord, I thought, I've been sandbagged. Lord, help thy unwilling, unworthy servant. I resolved never to go rabbit hunting with any policeman again.

Our first session did not go very well. Triangular therapy, not one on one. I checked the man's hearing. Normal. No organic abnormalities of the tongue or palate and good function. Articulation testing by naming pictures showed all the vowels and dipthongs to be produced adequately but the only good consonants were the /t/, /d/, /w/, /p/ and /n/. These he substituted for all others. Occasionally even these were omitted and only the vowel of the syllable was uttered. Generally he was pretty consistent in his errors on the same words. He could count up to a hundred: "uh," "too," "wee," and so on. He was also able to repeat five digits in his distorted fashion after an interval, so it wasn't a matter of short auditory memory span. When I asked him to repeat sentences of increasing length after my model and after a delay, he did so easily but unintelligibly, and when he repeated them again after an interval he said even a long sentence in the same way he had done before. One thing he couldn't do at all was to synthesize a series of isolated sounds. When I asked him to point to the picture of a sheep (sh...eee...p) he could not select it nor could he even integrate /n/ and /o/ to make the word "no"—one word which he could always say clearly. I asked his wife if she thought he understood what I was after, whereupon he replied at length. "He says sure he understands but he can't see that it makes any sense." I winced.

I then began to stimulate him strongly with isolated speech sounds, syllables and words, asking both of them to imitate me and to have him compare his utterance with hers. He could see no difference, she told me. When my model sound was /zzzz/ his first response was a single or repeated /d/. When I said that was wrong his wife prolonged the sound for him "ZZZZZZZ" again. William said "nnnn" and looked disgusted and he talked to her at length. "He says this is crazy stuff and why don't you start teaching him to talk?" she translated. William nodded strongly.

Chasing my brains all around in my skull and to gain time, I told them that first I would have to learn his language as she and the children had done. So I got out some pictures showing simple activities such as a boy running, a dog chewing a bone, a bird flying out of a nest, turned on the tape recorder and transcribed everything he said using the phonetic alphabet. I asked him to say each sentence twice and then I repeated as exactly as possible each of his utterances. I'm pretty sure I was able to imitate him pretty closely but each time he would say "No! No!" and then say it again for me to try again. And then he would yak excitedly but unintelligibly to his wife. She didn't translate. When I played back the tape it upset him greatly. He talked to her at some length. She shook her head. "He says that machine's no good." Mercifully, the long frustrating hour finally came to an end. I would see them again Friday, same time.

But I never did. The wife called me and said that William refused to come. He was happy the way he was. He didn't want to learn to talk right. "Besides, he said you weren't as smart as me and our kids if you couldn't learn to even talk like him or know what he means like we do, so how could you teach him?" I had no answer.

Programming Appropriate Reinforcements

Despite the previous examples, I have usually been able to keep my clients progressing in therapy by providing the appropriate reinforcements they required. Though I have religiously abstained from M&M's, I have been known to use single peanuts (on the theory that there is absolutely no satiation in one small peanut) with some of the children I served. I have often exploited not only the basic drive of hunger, but also those of thirst, sexual excitement, curiosity (the exploratory drive), and growth (self-actualization). Here is a short excerpt from a long play-by-play account of my work with a severe adult stutterer who lived with us for a year.*

The third group of activities presented the most difficulty and although he tried, Don was completely unable to follow a moment of stuttering with the prescribed silence, except occasionally with me or Lucy (his student clinician) and never in any other situation. Time pressure was evidently one of his major problems, as it is with most stutterers, but during these first two weeks Don seemed completely unable to cope with it. Lucy and I verbalized his distress for him and accepted the failures permissively, but it was evident that we would have to approach this problem more gradually. The other activities in this group showed increasing improvement. Occasionally, Don was able to integrate his fractured speech when he did not think he could. He reported instances of surprise when the expected stuttering did not occur or when it was shorter or milder than he had anticipated.

In the morning, Don was always starved. He would fix himself a good breakfast and then bring it into my study. I would then set up a bit of behavior to be rewarded by one small bit of egg or toast or one sip of coffee or orange juice. Often the food got cold before it was eaten and sometimes the conference period ended with much of it untouched. As Don gradually became more successful, however, we set up small quotas which had to be achieved before he took food. By this approximation to operant therapy (or a therapeutic infantile feeding situation, etc.), we attacked his eye closings, jaw jerks, abnormal mouth postures, tongue protrusions, the "um-but" starters and many other of the instrumental responses which formed so large a part of his abnormality. Significantly, we did not apply it to the tremors themselves. Occasionally, I would eat my breakfast with Don, and he could deprive me of a bite or sip by being able to say a word, phrase, or sentence without any of these reactions, even though stuttering occurred. He enjoyed these sessions.

I have also used sexual excitement, another primary reinforcer, to motivate some of my hornier clients. When I built my first speech clinic in the early thirties, I showed it to Dr. Bryng Bryngelson, of the University of Minnesota, with great pride. He courteously endured the tour of the therapy rooms and the laboratory before commenting, "Very nice and very unnecessary. All you really need is a davenport with a stutterer on one end and a pretty female therapist on the other." Anyway, I must confess that I have used this primary reinforcer at times, especially with post-adolescent stutterers who have often been sexually deprived. Here is an illustration:

*C. Van Riper, "Don: A Clinical Success." In H. Luper, ed., *Stuttering: Successes and Failures in Therapy*. Memphis: Speech Foundation of America, 1968.

We had a gangling freshman, who was weak and immature, and had an incredible variety of avoidance tricks. He seemed unable to make a real attempt on any feared word but had to postpone and filibuster until the pain of his long wait exceeded his fear of being unable to utter the word if he did try. Tremors traumatized him. He was also highly aware of his sexual needs but quite unable to attempt conversation with a girl because of his expectancy of rejection. At the time we also had a student therapist, a senior girl who had no objection to kissing boys in the interests of scientific research, so we enlisted her aid. The stutterer and this student therapist were placed before a mirror, and he was required to read some isolated words which he feared. For every three words on which he stuttered but did not avoid or postpone, she kissed him gaily and enthusiastically. After three or four of these very vivid experiences, he was absolutely unable to stutter. We then used consecutive material, which procured a few more kisses before the stuttering disappeared. Then the stutterer made some phone calls with the same result. The boy went back to his dormitory exhausted, but with his first free speech in years. He was back the next day seeking more of the same sort of therapy, but the experiment was over. He reported, however, that stuttering was never so feared again, and we were able to do considerably more direct therapy than previously. This sexual reward no doubt increased the approach gradient sufficiently to resolve some of his ambivalence.*

Here is another example of what strong motivation can do:

One day a very determined young lady phoned and demanded an immediate appointment for herself and her husband. This is what she said: "We were married yesterday after a whirlwind courtship. I had never heard my husband stutter before but he's been stuttering horribly ever since the ceremony. I love him but I'm not going to bed with a monster until I'm sure that he can be helped. Can you cure him? We have separate rooms at the Burdick Hotel and must see you immediately. Can we come up right now?"

Toujours l'amour, of course! The young man was indeed a very severe stutterer, gasping sequentially and compulsively until he blew himself up like a balloon, and only then could he utter the word he was trying to say. Pretty monosymptomatic too. I told his wife, who did all the talking, that I didn't know if I could help him but I'd try. She turned to her man and laid it on the line. "OK, we'll see. I'll give you three weeks before I go after an annulment. Meanwhile, you'll sleep alone." A pretty hard-nosed gal. Well, I've never had any stutterer work harder than that man, day and night. Self-therapy at its best. All I had to do was make a suggestion, explain a procedure or point out a goal. He improved very quickly and soon eliminated all the gasping. Never-

---

*From C. Van Riper, "Experiments in Stuttering Therapy." In Jon Eisenson, ed. *Stuttering: A Symposium*. New York: Harper and Row, 1958. Pp. 338–39.

theless, I was highly conscious of the calendar. Just before the three weeks were up, the man came in with a big cat-that-ate-the-canary grin on his face. "Well, Doc," he said, "I'm married at last, thanks to you." (And he stuttered on almost every word—but easily and without a gasp.)

Providing Faith and Trust

No clinician can rely on these primary reinforcers alone because his clients are not rats but very complex human beings. They are starved for many other things besides food, drink and sex. They hunger for acceptance, approval, companionship, faith and hope. When the clinician is the dispenser or fount of these, the client will work hard just to please him. Some have said that I have been an effective therapist because of my personal "charisma," whatever that nonsense word means. I do not believe it. Any ability to inspire or motivate my clients has been hard earned and hard learned. I have had to learn how to accept clients unconditionally, to set aside my own biases and negative feelings toward them, to react to their needs rather than to my own. A thousand experiences have taught me how to program appropriately my approvals and disapprovals. In this I am not unique. All good clinicians could tell the same story.

Yet perhaps my own personal history has made it easier for me to provide the genuine faith and hope these persons require, for when I look at the saddest specimen of humankind, I remember what a mess I once was, how hopeless and helpless. And I know that if I could have come out of that swamp of despair, anyone can! So it is a very real faith. Moreover, because I have seen many other human beings who have triumphed over adversities far worse than my own, and worse than those of this client before me, I always have a real hope that he can triumph too. So much for charisma!

These secondary reinforcers of approval and disapproval have value *only if our clients value us.* We cannot assume that they will. In fact, most of our clients come to us with much hidden skepticism, suspicion, or doubt. They have been hurt and betrayed by important people in their lives. You will have to earn their trust and regard, or your approvals will mean nothing. Why should they do what *you* want them to do? Why should they believe you? How can they be sure that you will not drop them if they put themselves in your hands?

Overtly or covertly, most of my clients have had to test me repeatedly before they could find satisfactory answers to these questions, and your clients will test you too. They do this testing in hundreds of ingenious ways, sometimes consciously, sometimes without being aware of the dynamics involved. Here are three dramatic illustrations of this testing.

Leonard was a high school senior who stuttered severely at times but who was usually fluent when he talked to his peers informally. He would not recite in school. He did not date girls. His mother, who referred him, said that Leonard was afraid to apply for a part-time job, and that when one was found for him, he refused to take it. A pretty miserable kid.

At first he was assigned to another member of our clinic staff. She came to me after the first two weeks and said, "This boy is not ready for therapy. Leonard has resisted doing almost everything I've suggested, or he has sabotaged, or at most put forth only a token effort. He hates me and hates himself. He's too much for me. Perhaps a man could get to him." So I said I'd work with Leonard.

After two weeks I was no more successful than she had been. Leonard sullenly refused to accept the invisible contract. He cooperated passively, if at all. One afternoon, after an especially thwarting session, I sat opposite him, thinking hard, chewing my pencil as I did so, and trying to think of some way to break through the invisible barriers that separated us so completely. When my secretary phoned to ask me to see her for a moment, I was relieved to have the interruption. After I returned to the inner office, I immediately sensed a marked change in Leonard's demeanour. He was tense, flushed, anxious—quite a change from the apathetic, sullen picture he had shown a few minutes before. "What now?" I thought, beginning again to chew the pencil, and I knew the answer immediately. While I was gone, the dirty little beast had put my pencil up his anus.

A wave of fury flooded me, as he sat there rigid. But then I did something impulsively I've been proud of ever since. I put the pencil back in my mouth and said quietly, "Now perhaps you can trust me, Leonard." The boy fled from the room and I beat the walls of the office with my fists for some time before I calmed down. That evening I drove over to Leonard's home and took him to the park for a long talk. I shall not tell what he sobbingly told me, but it was enough to explain why he could not trust me or anyone else, and why he hated himself and others. Then we had coffee and a pizza and became very close. Lord, how Leonard worked on his speech from that time on! And very successfully. I have never chewed a pencil since.

Fortunately, most of the testings the clinician encounters are less unpleasant than the one I have just recounted. The client will argue, or procrastinate, or lie or cheat, or attack you verbally. The experienced clinician does not resent these behaviors; they come with the job. They help the clinician know that he must demonstrate his competence and professionalism, that he must do more to create the needed solid relationship. But let me provide another sample of the testing process.

Margarita was the loveliest stutterer with whom I've ever worked. When she appeared for our first conference, I gasped.

Collecting myself, I began to ask the usual questions concerning her history. Margarita's response to my initial inquiry about her family was typically provocative: "I am a lineal descendant of the vestal virgins of Rome." She leaned forward as she said it and panted at me with half-closed eyes. The invitation was unmistakable. She wanted to play games. I steeled myself. "Did your grandfather stutter? Your grandmother? Your..." She broke into my questioning, "Doctor, do you like me? I like you... very much." She smiled gloriously and it was all I could do to keep my eyes off her heaving upper torso. Hastily, I terminated that first meeting, but I still remember her half-suppressed smile as Margarita gave me one last, long look before she undulated through the doorway.

I was ready for her at the time of our next therapy session. Coldly and efficiently, I outlined the course of therapy, described the terms of the invisible contract. I made it very clear that I was interested in her stuttering but not in her as a woman, that we had work to do. She tested me in every way possible—wept, flirted, teased. I remained adamant, the aloof professional clinician, interested but not taken in by her attempts to escape the need to confront and modify her stuttering.

Margarita had an interesting symptomatic picture. She alternately licked her lips and then puckered them, with little sucking noises when she blocked. A kissing stutterer. I drove her hard, demanding and insisting that she vary these behaviors. I made her duplicate her stuttering voluntarily. When she cried, I growled. When she refused to make a telephone call, I shamed her. I exhibited her before classes, providing a running commentary on her successes and failures. I programmed my approvals carefully so they were contingent upon *progress* toward the goals which had been set for her, and I was very sparing in administering them.

When Margarita became sexually provocative, I verbalized her motives as self-defeating resistance. Normally a warm and accepting therapist, with this girl I played a completely opposite role. I was almost brutal. At times I whipped her with my words. Margarita began to improve remarkably under the regime. Her speech became more and more fluent. She was interviewed on a radio program and only stuttered once. She tried out for a part in a Civic Theater production and was accepted. I began to hope that she might become free from her impediment.

Perhaps, as Margarita's recovery progressed so favorably, I let down my guard a little. Perhaps I smiled or looked at her legs instead of her mouth and she caught me doing so. I do not know. But one evening about 10 P.M., when I was sitting in my bachelor apartment smoking my pipe and reading a book, someone knocked on the door. It was Margarita. Her hair was touseled, her face was flushed and her eyes were wild. "F-f-f-forgive me for breaking in on you like this," she said in that low, husky, sexy voice, "But I have something very urgent to tell you and show you and I can't wait. Please! Please!" I nodded brusquely and gestured her to a chair, but she said, "May I use your bathroom for a minute first?" I indicated where she could find it.

When she reappeared she was naked as the dawn. She ran up to me, flung herself on my lap, threw her white arms around my neck and began kissing me passionately with a fury I had never known before and haven't known since. I flung her to the floor. "Get your clothes on and get the hell out of here!" I remember speaking the words coldly and deliberately. When she didn't go and came back to me, I turned her over my knee and spanked her bottom until it was rosy. Hard! It must have hurt but Margarita uttered no sound. I flung her to the floor again, and without a word she went to the bathroom, got her clothes and left. If she had tears in her eyes, I did not see them, for I was ostensibly back at my reading.

Oscar Wilde once said that the only way to get rid of a temptation was to yield to it. All I know is that the only temptations we remember are those we resisted. But I passed the test.

Lest I have given the impression that I do not possess my share of the frailty which is common to all of us, I should tell you about Hal. I failed his testing and lost him forever. Hal's problem was severe hypernasality, for which we could find no organic cause. His mother also showed some of the same voice quality, though it was not as abnormal as Hal's, and I had wondered if some abnormal identification existed between the two of them. I never did find out because I lost my temper. Here's how it happened.

Soon after I began to work with Hal, he underwent a religious conversion and became a member of a small, far-out fundamentalist sect. Usually, when a client is in any process of fundamental change, we can take advantage of that moment of arousal to change some of the client's speech patterns. Unfortunately, Hal became very evangelistic and focused his proselyting efforts on me. Now, I admit that I'm sure my soul could profit from some saving, but not from an unctuous new saint. Besides, he had zeroed in, as many clients seem to have an uncanny ability to do, on one of my Achille's heels, on an area of real vulnerability. I have never been very secure in my religious beliefs or disbeliefs.

Anyway, my job was to help Hal get and maintain a voice free from that constant nasal whine. Our sessions produced little progress, with most of the time spent in defining my role and defending myself against his challenges. Often I felt more like the client than the clinician. Hal began to send notes to my home saying that he was praying for me. He presented me with a Bible. Finally, one day he barged into my office unexpectedly while I was making an important phone call and got down on his knees, praying loudly and whiningly for my black soul. After I hung up and contemplated him for a few moments, I noticed him watching me carefully under his half-closed, pious eyelids. So I picked him up by the collar and literally booted him out of the door and part way down the hall. Then I returned to my office, shocked and ashamed of what I had done. What a therapist I have turned out to be!

Whenever I have found myself over-reacting to a client's behavior, I know that it must be pointing to a basic weakness in me, and that it is time for me to analyze my past to discover what it is. Here are some of the old memories that flooded back:

When I was eight or nine, a little boy, I became terribly concerned about my own stuttering, for often I could not utter a sound and grotesque facial and body contortions were beginning to appear. Finally, in desperation, I asked my mother what I could do and she told me to pray to God for deliverance from my impediment. So I prayed. Not just at bedtime either, but every chance I got— even in the outhouse. However, I never prayed aloud because even when I talked to myself I stuttered abjectly. I also tried to be very good and not to hit my little brother or to spill any milk or to shoot the cows with my BB-gun. In fact, my behavior was so exemplary that my father pulled me to one side one day and asked me what the hell was wrong with me. He looked at my tongue, examined my feces, and felt my pulse before giving me a compound cathartic in the belief that I must have worms. Not only did I go to Sunday School willingly, which was a marked contrast to my usual behavior, but I even begged them to let me stay for church. My grandmother approved the change and slipped me a stick of the striped peppermint candy from the jar she hid in her spare corset. Grandma Van always gave me some when I asked her to read to me from her little black Bible.

Well, as I said, I prayed hard and long and eloquently for days and months. Every morning when I awoke I would hope that the miracle had happened and that my stuttering was gone. (I think most young severe stutterers feel the same way.) I remember well one time when I thought it really had disappeared. I talked all the way through breakfast without blocking and ran out to tell our horse Billy that at last I could speak, only to find myself mute and struggling again. I remember weeping there in the stall and wondering why God who, Gramma said, heard every sparrow chirp, seemed unable to hear my pleas. Or if he had heard, why had he refused to help a troubled little boy? I finally decided that it was because I wasn't praying out loud, so I tried that too. It was pretty miserable though, for I stuttered on almost every word I said to Him and I knew it didn't sound very good. I used to imagine the same scowl on His face that appeared on my father's when he had to listen to my stuttering. Sometimes I would block so hard I had to quit praying because I was crying too much.

About this time my other grandma, who was very proud because I had learned to read books at the age of three, sent me one entitled "A Child's History of Ancient Greece." It was full of the tales of Greek mythology and I devoured it hungrily. The one that hit me hardest, though, was about Ajax on the mountain top, baring his breast and daring Zeus to strike him down with his thunderbolts.

For some reason, that tale of man's ineffable courage in challenging the gods had a great impact on me. I could not forget it. It reverberated in my thoughts like a perseverative tune. And it was probably because of Ajax that one weekday afternoon after school I crept into the always-open doors of the Methodist Episcopal Church and committed the ultimate heresy.

I'm not sure that I can communicate the feelings of that little boy as he tremblingly tip-toed down the long aisle between the empty pews and confronted the altar and that great arch behind it where he thought God dwelt. The boy was shaking so hard he could hardly unbutton his jacket, but he finally did so and then said quaveringly, "Dear God, I've asked you but I still can't talk right. I ask you now. Cure my stuttering." There was only silence. And then the boy looked up at the crest of the arch and cried, "I don't think you're there. I don't think you're you. There ain't no God." Sobbing, he ran down the aisle and out of the tall doors as though the devil himself were grabbing at his flying jacket. He hid in the haymow until suppertime, waiting for the thunderbolt.

If I remember right, the boy was covertly feeling rather proud of himself—like Ajax—until suddenly the terrible thought hit him that, of course, he had been able to get away with it on Thursday. But come Sunday, then God would get him. That's when *He* was in *His* house.

The boy did not pray that night nor the other nights till the Sabbath came, but he worried plenty and cried himself to sleep. On Sunday he *was* sick and took the castor oil and calomel without protest. Another week went by and he was sick again on Sunday and then another week. But this time, his mother literally dragged him to church. A dark day with black scudding clouds! The boy's terror made him clutch his mother there in the pew with both arms. Even if he was bad, *she* was good, and God wouldn't want to hurt *her*. She could not quiet the boy's shaking and sobbing. Thunder in the distance, then rain spattering on the roof of the church as the sermon droned on. Finally, there came a tremendous flash of light and the biggest bang in the world shook the wooden building.

The preacher and half of the congregation were on their knees but the little boy was under the pew with both his hands over his head, waiting, waiting. His mother picked him up and, recognizing the utter terror, took him from the service and brought him home. As they went out of the church door, it was clear what had happened. The lightning bolt had struck a large maple tree in the churchyard, splitting it into strips. The boy's mother said, more to herself than to him, "There'll be less sinning among the congregation this next week." The boy said only two words: "HE missed!" and he didn't stutter on either of them. One thunderbolt was enough to waste on one small boy and so somehow he was comforted.

It is very difficult to know what runs through the minds of children with severe speech problems. They can't or won't tell you of their hurts, often because the telling hurts them all over again. Clinicians must be aware of this or they will fail to discern the hidden emotional part of the handicap that often must be dealt with if therapy is to be successful.

But I was attempting to explain why I had behaved so unclinically with Hal, why I had been so vulnerable to his testing me by trying to convert me. The incident just recounted hardly seemed sufficient to explain my sudden fury or why I kicked him. Evidently some deeper probing was needed. What else in my history might have more significance in accounting for my wretched behavior? Suddenly, I remembered a revival meeting experience in which a traveling evangelist created a terrible scene as he vainly tried for a long time to get me to come up to the altar and confess my sins publicly. (I not only couldn't think of any real sins but I didn't want to display my stuttering.) I also remembered a young clergyman who befriended me when I needed friends badly and then tried to assault me homosexually. And other unpleasant memories connected with religion! All this self-probing yielded some understanding of why I reacted so badly to Hal's behavior, but it is explanation not justification.

I suspect that I shall always be somewhat vulnerable in the religious area, but I'm sure that another Hal would not be able to evoke such a response from me. The best armor is always forged from understanding. I can think of at least five better ways of responding to his testing, but alas! I will never have the opportunity to use them with him. I missed my chance to help Hal at that moment and even now, twenty years later, that troubles me. I was unworthy of his trust.

THE CLINICIANS SKILLS

Although the client's perception that he can trust the integrity of the therapist is basic, he also needs a clinician who can understand him deeply. Some of my clients have felt terribly alienated from society; most of them have felt helplessly alone far too often. It is always difficult to know another person, but I have found repeatedly that many of my mistakes were due to my insensitivity to the client's needs and feelings. Just one brief example:

A young Chinese man came from Hong Kong with a very severe stuttering problem. Though he spoke English fairly well, at first I could not read his body language at all. I just could not tune in to Chang. After I had misinterpreted his facial expressions, body postures, and gestures too many times in a row, I studied him hard and long and finally managed to be able to occasionally translate them with some fidelity. I found that if Chang smiled or giggled, it meant that he was deeply embarrassed. If he nodded his head up and down, it meant only that he understood, not that he agreed. If Chang smiled and sucked air through his teeth, it meant that he was completely rejecting what I was suggesting. If he looked away, it meant that he was thoughtfully considering doing it. Even so, we couldn't understand each other on any but a superficial level. Since I could not identify with him, he couldn't identify with me either. There was no leverage. One special problem was that Chang absolutely refused to examine or analyze the stuttering behaviors he had come from so far away to eliminate.

When I brought out a mirror so he could see how he stuttered, Chang bolted from the therapy room and did not return for two weeks. After three months of this frustration, I went to our Oriental cafe and asked the proprietor, a friend for many years, to help me. He told me something that I had not gained from any of the books on Chinese culture that I had been studying: that one of the basic Chinese values was to live so as to be a credit to oneself, to one's family and to one's ancestors. Stuttering was a very disgraceful act, completely unacceptable. The proprietor told me that there were two kinds of face (pride), *lien* and *mien,* one referring to the self and family, and the other to the ancestors. "When Chang stutters, a thousand ancestors turn over in their graves and lie face down." Anyway, that's what my friend told me, and it led to some real progress in therapy.

I told Chang what I had learned and he agreed, or I thought he did. Then I videotaped him as he was making some phone calls and stuttering badly. Next, this hierarchy was developed for Chang's viewing his stuttering tape when maintaining a relaxed state and *while being completely alone:* (1) Watching it through half closed eyes with the sound off; (2) watching with eyes closed but with the sound turned on; (3) with eyes open and with sound; (4) counting all stutterings; (5) categorizing them into different classes of stuttering behavior; (6) imitating each moment of stuttering simultaneously with the image on the screen; (7) stuttering differently, smoothly and without tension, whenever he saw a bit of his old stuttering, but doing it in unison with his screen image.

It took Chang two weeks of working five hours a day alone by himself before he completed the program and was ready for intensive therapy, first with me and then in outside speaking situations. I'm sure that had I not come to understand how necessary it was for him to "save face," we would have failed abjectly. All severe stutterers find it hard to confront their stuttering behaviors objectively, but at least they don't have a thousand ancestors turning face down in their graves when they do so.

Providing Hope

Clinicians must also learn how to arouse hope. It is a very powerful motivating force. The client cannot have much hope if the clinician has little. Somehow I've always been able to find enough favorable prognostic signs in the sorriest of my clients to believe that he can be helped, but you often have to hunt for these signs. You often have to blow hard on the embers before hope will flare.

In the forty-five years that I spent in the vineyard of speech pathology, I have worked with many individuals who had articulation disorders. Usually we tend to think that these problems are easier to solve than those of language, voice or fluency, but some of those that I have encountered have tested my competence to its limits. With some I have failed abjectly. One of these was the young son of a fellow faculty member whose only error was the addition of an /i/ vowel to every final /r/ sound. He would say "The berry is scaried of firey" for "The bear is scared of fire." I did my utmost and so did the boy, but at the end of six months of almost daily therapy, he still could not keep that intrusive /i/ from following the /r/ in his spontaneous speech. I checked up on him six years later and the error was gone. He said he'd outgrown it. Ach!

The various kinds of lisps are not usually troublesome, but one adult with a bad lateral emission of air on the /s/ and /z/ sounds (with a bubble of saliva in it) never was able to transfer the perfect sibilants he finally could achieve in nonsense syllables or words to the rest of his speech. He tried hard and so did I, and I still don't know why we failed. In other persons, some of the /r/ semivowel errors have been equally resistant to change or transfer, and so I have always had a close feeling of fellowship with my colleagues in the public schools who must tackle these problems daily.

Nevertheless, there have been some successes, too. One of our local ministers told me of Ruth E., a woman of forty, who had stopped talking for several years after a stroke had resulted in a partial left hemiplegia. Though Ruth's left eyelid drooped, the left side of her face sagged and she seemed unable to move her left hand or arm, I found no evidence of dysphasia. She understood everything she read or heard and she communicated effectively in writing. But she was mute. Indeed, she was reconciled to being speechless for the rest of her life.

This didn't make sense. There was no language disability, no paralysis of the vocal folds. Surely she could produce sound or at least be able to whisper. But she didn't! Evidently her pencil and paper had come to be her vocal folds. Neurosis? Hysterical mutism? She just didn't seem to fit those patterns. I could detect no secondary gains.

When Ruth's mouth was examined, however, I immediately noticed that her tongue was asymmetrical in size, the left half looking shrunken and withered, and that, when in a resting position, it was also pulled away from the midline toward the cheek. Nevertheless she could lift it, though slowly and clumsily, to make contact with the spots I touched with a swabstick. Contacts were searched for and found on the soft palate, hard palate, upper gum and upper teeth, but she could not seem voluntarily to be able to protrude the tongue between the teeth. When Ruth tried to do so, the tongue curled to one side within the mouth. Functionally she had only half a tongue, but surely that was enough. How could I convince her to believe that she could use it—that she need not be speechless all the rest of her life?

I remembered Michael J. Flynn, a plumber, whom Dr. Goldstein had presented to an early A.S.H.A. convention long before. Mike had no tongue at all—or rather just the stump of one—yet he could speak very intelligibly. Somewhere in the clinic I still had a recording of Michael J. Flynn, and a picture of his mouth with the little bulge of tissue that once had been his tongue. I would try to use both to teach Ruth to speak again. She had to have hope.

But how to do it? I debated within myself the choice of strategies. Finally

I decided to speak bluntly. "Ruth," I said, "I can teach you to talk again so you don't have to spend the rest of your life with that pencil and paper. I know you had a stroke and that part of your tongue is still paralyzed, but there is no reason why you cannot produce voice or whisper. Indeed, I know you can, for I heard you cough *aloud* the other day, and also make some sound when you cleared your throat. I think I know what happened, my friend. After the stroke, when you did try to speak, you found you couldn't move your tongue in the old ways and the sounds you tried to say were all garbled or some of them you could not make at all. And so you quit trying. It's quite natural that you would. The tragedy of these last three years, though, is that you didn't know that half a tongue is enough, more than enough to be able to talk with. You've got to learn how to use it, of course, but that's my job."

I still have the note she wrote me? "I'd like to believe you but I can't." It was then that I showed her the picture of Michael J. Flynn's mouth and had her listen to his recording. She was impressed and eager to begin right then, but I told her we'd start the next day.

Why did I desire that postponement? I am not sure. Who knows always why we do what we do in therapy? Perhaps I felt some time was needed for my words to sink in, to have impact. Perhaps time was required for her motivation to grow. Perhaps I needed the time myself to plan how to get Ruth to produce that first vocalized speech after three years of muteness. I knew I would have to be careful. If that first utterance were too garbled, the hope would fade quickly.

The next day, using the mouth shaping and touching techniques of the motokinesthetic method, and with strong auditory stimulation, I got Ruth to utter the words "I" and "am," then the sentence "I am talking." (She said "todding") in a husky, rusty voice. Then the flood of tears came and I had to hunt for the Kleenex in my desk drawer. The subsequent therapy was prolonged and often difficult, for we had to work on almost every sound except the vowels, searching for the compensatory movements necessary to produce it. But the therapy was also highly enjoyable for both of us. Ruth never learned to make a really acceptable /r/ sound, except perhaps in its consonant form, so I said to her, "What's wrong with having a Southern accent, honey child?" and we let it go at that. Later she even returned to work. So once again I learned that you can do almost anything if you think you can.

Understanding Our Client

All Clinicians should also train themselves in the subtle skills that enable them to sense the hidden feelings of their clients. These are not to be found in textbooks or classrooms. They must be mastered in the situations of intimate human encounter. Some of my students and clients have felt that I had an uncanny ability to read their thoughts—and at times I have indeed experienced something akin to clairvoyance—but only after I had observed and identified closely with the person long enough. I hate to give an example of this because it always sounds fraudulent. In any event, I do not feel that this ability is God- or devil-given. It is the result of very careful observation, uninhibited inference making, and the calculation of probabilities. It comes through *empathy*.

Because this ability to understand another human being is so useful in therapy, I trained myself for many years to develop it in myself and in my students. I learned the skill of shadowing the speech of others, saying what they said at almost the same time they said it. First, I did this aloud when listening to speakers on the radio, then covertly when listening to others. I tried to match not only the words, but the tempo, voice inflections and pauses as well. One can also learn to "shadow" the gestures, postures, and movements of other people almost as actors do in learning a role.

I also worked hard to train myself in the psychotherapist's art of *reflecting*—being able to express the real meaning of what your client is trying or wanting to say in your own words. I constantly tried to finish (covertly) the unfinished sentences that my client left hanging uncompleted so I might follow his chains of association. I endeavored to predict his responses, to anticipate what he would do or say next. In short, I tried for the moment to be that other person. Oh, the failures I had in this self-training—thousands of them—usually because I was out of tune, but the failures themselves led to more understanding. Of course, each new client presented a new problem in empathy, but gradually they became easier for me to read. However, adolescent girls and boys have continued to baffle me all my days—perhaps because my stuttering prevented me from having a normal adolescence. These adolescents have, as did Chang, a different culture. But let me tell you what happened in Peoria.

Long ago, when I was just beginning my career, I had gone there to participate in a workshop, had contributed my nonsense but had to stay over another day before returning home. And I was bored. Perhaps you don't know Peoria. After you've looked at the window displays at the stores ten times, you might as well go back to your hotel. There was a wonderful little monologue in the old play "Lightning" that said it best: "How come I got married? Well, I was in Peoria. I was in Peoria Friday, Saturday, Sunday and Monday. It rained every day in Peoria. So I got married!" Unfortunately, I was already married and, reduced to the desperation of reading the ads in the local paper, I came across one that announced that a carnival had come to town. So I got a cab and hied myself thither. The merry-go-round did not recapture my youth and I soon tired of watching the freaks watching the freaks in the sideshows. I was about to leave when I spied a fortune-teller's tent. Madame Rosie, a big-bellied wanton in kerchief and red-flowered draperies, presided. Did I want the crystal ball of Oom, or the tea leaves, or the reading of palms? Five dollars, two dollars, one dollar? I chose the last of these delights, but told the Madame that I would pay her five dollars instead if I felt she had done a good job. The challenge impressed Rosie. "OK, gimme yer mitt!" she ordered.

Then followed a torrent of verbalization, ceaselessly flowing, as Madame Rosie alternately scanned my hand and face. It continued for at least five minutes before she stopped and said, "Gimme the five bucks!" I paid it without a murmur because in all that monologue she had hit the nail on the head so many times I was astonished in spite of myself. She told me that I was some kind of a professor, probably a psychologist; that I was married and had one child, a girl; that I was having a hard time financially; that I had been brought up among foreigners; that I had had some severe emotional problems centered about talking and had been hospitalized for a time; that others thought me a bit askew and odd; that I liked to gamble and was a poor loser but a worse winner; and that I hated Peoria and wanted to get the hell out of there. All these statements were absolutely true. I'm sure that there were others that weren't, but I couldn't remember them. Madame Rosie retrieved her gum from under the crystal ball and grinned as I sat there thinking. "And right now, you're wondering how I do it, hey?" True again! "And now you're wondering if I'll tell you how I do it if you give me five more bucks, Sonny. Well, I won't. Professional secret. Anyway, you can't afford it." True!

"Madame Rosie," I said respectfully, "you are indeed very good but I think I've figured out how you do it. First of all, you aren't a damned bit interested in the lines on my hand; it's my face and body that you were watching. And the first thing you do in all that patter of yours is to make statements, very obvious and true ones about ordinary things so you can see how I show my agreement. You check my positive responses. Then you do the same for the negative ones, saying something like 'On a cool day like this' (when you know it's hotter than hell and I'll disagree) to find out how I say *no* with my facial expressions or body postures. You figure out how I say 'yea' and 'nay' to whatever you are saying. When you get a yea, you finish the sentence, but if you see a negative response, you shift to something else. And when you get a hot lead, you follow it up, getting yea after yea. You talk so much and you talk so fast and cover so many areas, you're bound to hit pay dirt sooner or later. And you're sure good!"

Madame Rosie looked me over, thinking hard. "Sonny," she said, "you've hit it pretty close. I learned the jag from my hubby, the Great Ozymandias, and he was the best one in the business. I've been on the circuit a long time and you're the first that ever figured it out. How about joining the act? I'll teach you all I know, all the tricks. We could really pull in the swag. Anyway, I need a man in the act for the dames. They're too suspicious of a woman. But you'll have to raise a beard and take off them glasses. It's a good life, Sonny. See the country. Suckers everywhere. How about it?'' God help me, I was tempted for a moment until Rosie took out her gum, contemplated it, and put it back under Oom. So I thought of my beautiful wife and child, bade a regretful farewell and went back to Peoria.

I never forgot my lesson, however, and have worked hard to become alert to the body language of anyone who may play an important part in my life. I check for their yeas and nays and follow the positive leads wherever they take me. I doubt that I will ever be as good as the Great Ozymandias, but I'm still trying. All I know is that the skill has become important to me in understanding my clients. It helps me help them. All clinicians should acquire it. Indeed, I have found only one drawback: after the men in the Kalamazoo Cultural Uplift Society, our poker group, finally figured out why I was winning consistently, they insisted that if I wanted to play I couldn't open my mouth, except for a snort from the brown bottle.

Success and Failure

I do not wish to imply that my empathetic batting average was ever very high; certainly it has never been high enough to please me. Human beings are often hidden under many layers of veils and defenses. Moreover, they do not want these uncovered, lest they see themselves naked in the mirror of your eyes. (Because I respect these feelings I do my scanning as quietly and covertly as I can.) All I know is that when I have been completely unable to have any kind of close clinical identification with a client, I have usually failed to help him, no matter what methods I used or how hard I tried. I submit, a bit reluctantly, an example.

I have had a number of stutterers with whom I have consistently failed, despite strenuous efforts to help them. They seem to me to have certain characteristics in common, and the person I have called Melinda is quite representative of this group. At the termination of therapy, they were stuttering as frequently and severely as they were at its beginning. Follow-ups were difficult to achieve, but in those I was able to contact several years later, the disorder had shown no change. I have repeatedly reviewed their case folders and my clinical notes to try to comprehend the reasons for their intransigence or my ineptitude. Perhaps the present analysis will be more successful than those which preceded it. Anyway!

When she first enrolled in our program of intensive therapy, Melinda was a very attractive person—one of the most beautiful women I have known. She also stuttered more consistently and with greater frequency than almost any stutterer I have met. On the average, about 90% of her words showed abnormality, and this frequency rate did not vary much from situation to situation.

Though occasionally she might say a phrase or short sentence without repetitions, only once did I hear her be completely fluent for several minutes. Melinda was making a phone call and did not know anyone was near, and she was giving some girl friend billy blue hell. For almost five minutes she talked freely and with much profanity and vulgarity. When I walked in, her voice and speech changed, and the stuttering reappeared.

Melinda's stuttering was monosymptomatic, consisting of rapid syllabic repetitions using the schwa vowel. I once counted 28 on a single word with an inspiration taken partway through the sequence, but the number of repetitions closely averaged about seven or eight. Melinda was the only stutterer I have ever heard to repeat compulsively the final unaccented syllable of a polysyllabic word. Often, if by chance she would happen to say several words in a row without stuttering, I would hear her return to the same phrase or last word thereof and repeat its first or accented syllable. She cancelled her fluent words by stuttering.

Another characteristic of the repetitions was the lack of accompanying tremors or fixations. The repeated syllables were not very regular in their tempo. They started slowly, then became faster. Once started, they ran on, uninterrupted until the word was uttered. No rise in pitch accompanied the accelerating repetitions, nor was there any tension or struggle. She just buh-buh-buh-buh-buh-bounced and bounced interminably. Interestingly enough, though she reported situation fears, she had few phonemic or word fears. Melinda could not remember the sounds of words on which she had stuttered, even when an accounting was requested immediately after the conclusion of an utterance. This seeming detachment (or a real one) apparently insulated her from the confrontation of her abnormal speech behavior. She could not sense it, remember it or stop it. When a mirror was placed before her, she shut her eyes or they became glazed. When I played back a recording, she would just laugh. "That sure sounds silly, doesn't it?" she said, but without emotion. I never could get Melinda to accept her stuttering objectively. She gaily and easily admitted that she was a stutterer, in fact "a stuttering mess," but the comment always seemed perfunctory.

Melinda showed very few avoidances. She entered all ordinary speaking situations; she telephoned, interrupted, argued. She also enrolled in several classes in public speaking, much to the distress of her instructors. One of them told me, "My God, keep those stutterers out of my hair. That Melinda girl tortures all of us. She takes up more class time than any three other students combined. If she weren't so sweet and beautiful and courageous, I'd kick her out."

Melinda showed few postponement tricks antecedent to her repetitions, no "ah's" or "ums" as starters, no circumlocution or substitutions. She plunged directly into her repetitive utterance without any sign of faltering. Another characteristic, perhaps significant, was that she showed no reaction immediately after her moments of stuttering, no pauses, no flushing—nothing! The basic prosody was unaffected except for the reduced inflection. She spoke a stuttering language.

Melinda always maintained excellent eye contact. She had beautiful jet black eyes, and she kept them upon you constantly, almost hypnotically. She seemed always to be scanning you—testing, testing, testing. The intensity of her gaze increased at the moments of stuttering. At the same time, however, she smiled a bittersweet smile. Not much humor in it—just a beautiful, brave little girl smiling away the monsters and ghosts. Most people did not see her testing eyes. They saw only her smile. Melinda had, in fact, received very few consistent penalties for her stuttering. She always seemed to have girl friends and acquaintances in quantity, though the relationships seemed unstable. Melinda's brave little smile reduced others into wanting to mother or take care of her. "She seems so brave and sweet," one of her housemothers said. I found Melinda as tough as leather and hard as corundum. She was not helpless at all. She was one of the most controlling females I have ever met—and that constitutes more than a few. Even her whims were of iron.

In the course of my career I have come to expect resistance from my clients as part of the therapy process—indeed, as a very essential part. Too much compliance always worries me. Anyone who has stuttered for years has incorporated the disorder into the very bones of his personality. There is rendering of soul flesh when one begins to remove it. We protect and seek to maintain all equilibria, even those uncomfortable ones which distress us. But Melinda fought me to the ground whenever I sought to get her to modify her stuttering. Very intelligent, she constantly outwitted me. To cite but one example, once I had contrived to get her to promise to appear before a group of speech therapists at a professional meeting and to describe and comment upon each moment of stuttering she experienced. She was committed. I had blocked—so I thought—every other exit. I took her to the meeting in my car. Five minutes before the meeting, after going to the ladies' room, she told me she could not go through with it. Her face was covered with a reddish purple rash; her eyes were almost swollen shut. Even her arms and hands were puffed and discolored. All that had happened in five minutes. I kicked myself for my stupidity in hoping that she finally had been brought to the point of accepting her stuttering as a problem.

As I look back on all those daily sessions (and I worked with her daily for a year), I wonder why I persisted. It was probably professional vanity. Melinda and her ilk have taught me professional humility. I now think she enjoyed the whole business. She played the game skillfully, always giving me enough intermittent hope to allow the game to continue. I believe she knew she would win. She played games with me. Were they sexual games? If so, she covered the dynamics skillfully. Certainly there were no sign of flirtation in her behavior. Could it have been a latent homosexuality, using the therapy room as the battlefield against a male therapist? Melinda dated several boys regularly and evidently enjoyed them, and they her. I interviewed one of the boys who had taken her out repeatedly, and he said she was fun but not very warm. "I always have the feeling she's watching herself and me. She's not there." For two months I administered therapy through an attractive woman therapist. No difference.

In my review of Melinda's file, I find that my clinical notes on our therapy sessions are sketchy, much more so than those of the other stutterers I have served. This was due in part to the fact that Melinda revealed very little about herself despite my probings. She was an incredibly expert conversational fencer. Her lie score on the MMPI was high, and I never really trusted any information she offered. I know that she often did not tell the truth about her self-therapy assignments. In our sessions together, however, she was usually quite cooperative in a token way, always doing a little but never enough. At times she would report a glorious triumph in a situation which I could never check upon. A few "facts" may be given here. Melinda was an only child of wealthy parents. Very precocious physical and social development. Began to stutter suddenly on school entrance into kindergarten at five years. Stuttering was severe and frequent from the first. "My parents tell me it's the same now as it was then." No stuttering in the family. A pleasant home. The usual summer camps and travels. Excellent educational achievement. Accepted socially despite her stuttering. Parents had sought all sorts of professional help. "Finally, they just gave up on me" she reported. Melinda had her own car at college, plenty of money, and she dressed attractively.

The reader will of course be wondering why I accepted such a client for speech therapy or continued to work with her so long. I do not think it was just because she was beautiful, but rather because her stuttering was so consistent and frequent. No one should have to go through life talking like that. All the patterning of behaviors indicated neurosis and I recognized this very soon, but I have always considered the particular kind of speech therapy I practice to be essentially a psychotherapy, too. Most severe stutterers show some signs of neurosis, though it is usually an expectancy neurosis. In contrast, Melinda could not be described as phobic by any stretch of the word. She had very little expectancy. I could find no evidence of profit from her symptoms, though possibly they might have served as a defense against a latent homosexuality. To check this, I referred Melinda to a psychiatrist colleague for whom I have the profoundest respect. After a series of interviews, he assured me that no primary neurosis existed. Also, Melinda told me that a famous psychoanalyst in Boston had explored the matter for several months and had refused to accept her for deep analysis, saying that she did not need it. It is my feeling now that Melinda fooled them, too. Perhaps I am merely trying to salvage my own professional self-respect, but I'm pretty well convinced that her stuttering was symptomatic of a deep primary neurosis. When finally I confessed my inability to continue therapy for another single session and confronted her with this diagnosis, Melinda said with that same brave, sweet smile, "Oh, I'm sorry too, Dr. Van. I had such hopes in you. But please, Dr. Van, you must not let this experience make you feel incompetent or discouraged." Damn her hide!*

I deplore that last statement because, of course, I was probably projecting the irritation I felt with myself. It was my professional hide that I was damning. Usually, when I have failed I have learned something important that I can put to good use with some other client. But in my head I have replayed my encounters with Melinda as a chess master replays his game, and although I can see a few things I would do differently were I to have another client like her, they are not sufficient. Melinda was right. I just wasn't competent enough. I did not understand her at all.

---

*This tale was previously published in The Speech Foundation of America's booklet *Successes and Failures in Stuttering Therapy* and is reprinted by permission.

THE REWARDS
OF
THERAPY

I always hate to feel that I have not had any impact at all on a client, for of all the rewards of therapy, the feeling of *meaningfulness* is the greatest. Fortunately, experiences such as those with Melinda have been rare. There were other failures, as some of my earlier anecdotes have revealed, but usually at worst they were partial failures, and a partial failure is also a partial success. Although I was not able to solve the problem completely, I knew that the person was probably better off for having become involved in therapy. For example, several clients who failed to achieve the goals of therapy then went elsewhere to get the relief they did not find with me, or found it by themselves. In these instances I feel that I at least helped them solve many problems that would otherwise have thwarted their efforts. Lose some, win some, but do your damndest!

Opportunities for Personal Growth

Besides this all-important feeling of meaningfulness, therapy brings to one's life the great satisfactions of personal growth. All of us must grow or we die. Almost every client I have served has helped me sense this personal growth. One of those who had a real impact on me was Abdul, who found our clinic because one of my books had been translated into Arabic.

Abdul, a stutterer from Arabia, was one of my most difficult cases. Almost as old as I was, good-looking in a somewhat sinister way, he stuttered viciously, hissing and spitting like a cobra. He trusted no one and his suspicion almost bordered upon paranoia. When I smiled, he sought an evil, morbid explanation for that smile. When I cleared my throat, he interpreted the act as suppressed nausea. Abdul guarded his past history vigilantly, and only the most skillful probing elicited such neutral facts as his age and home address. Nevertheless, I persisted, and gradually the man and his problem began to show their outlines.

Part of the difficulty was due to the treatment Abdul had received in Arabia from almost everyone he met. All of his countrymen had rejected him as though he had leprosy. From childhood, strangers would flee his presence when they heard him stutter. Mothers would curse him and snatch their children away lest they become infected. Clerks would spit at him and refuse to serve him. Despised by his fellow students, and confronted by constant obstacles placed in his way by his teachers, only his exceptional intelligence enabled him to win a precarious overseas scholarship to do research at a southern university in this country. Somehow he managed to find some devious means for justifying a four-month leave from his studies to "cure his stuttering" at our clinic.

Unfortunately, the sort of therapy that I practice requires the stutterer to confront his stuttering so that he can modify it. Abdul wanted to be rid of his impediment without this confrontation. He could not bear to listen to it on the tape recorder; he would not look at his grimaces and contortions in the mirror. He didn't even want to think about it or discuss it. "Cure me!" he demanded. "But don't bring up the subject of stuttering!" All stutterers show some of this denial of the problem and they resist the necessary task of specifying the behaviors they must alter and extinguish, but Abdul's resistance was immense and total.

Seeking ways to overcome his obstinate refusal to examine his stuttering behaviors, I explored the beliefs of his culture concerning the disorder, even reading the entire Koran from cover to cover along with various other commentaries on Arabic culture. I studied Arabian art, immersed myself in the literature and history and found it fascinating. One very important insight occurred. In the religion of Islam, *Allah,* God, is in you incarnate when you are highly aware and in command of yourself, but *Al Kohol,* the devil, is in you when you are not. That is why the Mohammedans are not supposed to drink any liquor, and that is why epileptics and persons with cerebral palsy are so instantly rejected. Their seizures and contortions reveal the visible presence of Satan in all of his evil threat. That is why Abdul had been rejected so severely. When he saw his stuttering in the clinic mirror, Abdul saw Al Kohol in the flesh, his own flesh. No wonder I couldn't get him to confront his stuttering behaviors.

After two months, there had been no progress whatsoever, and Abdul's time was running short. In some desperation I took him along with me on a week's speaking trip to several southern universities, and on the way I revealed my interest in his religion and shyly suggested that he seek to convert me to his faith. As you can imagine, he was instantly and thoroughly suspicious of my motives, but when I kept quoting the Koran and showed how much I had read about his culture, he was impressed in spite of himself. When I joined him every morning on his little prayer rug outside the rear of our motel, facing east with our rears raised high and I chanted "Allah, il Allah. Akhbar!" even louder than he did, he became almost convinced that I was indeed seeking *The Way*.

And in a sense, I was. I've never had any real religion of the formal sort and have envied the serenity of those who do. Moreover, I have witnessed profound changes in the personalities of persons who suddenly found a faith. I have been amazed at the strength shown by truly religious cancer victims as they endured their last agonies. And I have never been able to forget my Aunt Nell, whose face at 80 was the most beautiful face I have ever seen. Her life had been full of tragedy: a difficult husband, two sons killed, a host of miseries. And yet she could say again and again that her life had been a wonderful one. "Every morning when I get up, I ask the Lord what wonderful thing he has in store for me that day, and, you know, never once has he failed me." She was certain that God held her in his arms.

As I told Abdul about my search and my hunger for a religious faith, he began to believe that I was somewhat sincere in my desire to understand the religion of his Prophet Mohammed. Anyway, he began to expound and prose-lyte, and when he did a curious thing happened: most of his stuttering disap-peared. When I pointed this out to Abdul he said, "Of course, it is Allah speaking, not me! Allah does not stutter. Allah, il Allah, Akhbar!" I joined the chant automatically but I was thinking hard. How could I keep Allah inside Abdul's mouth or skin and keep Al Kohol out?

I remembered James Hunt, an old therapist for stutterers, whose book was published in 1869. In it he said that the secret of his success in therapy was that he made his stammerers speak consciously as others speak uncon-sciously. The prescription seemed expressly designed for Abdul. If I could get him to be highly aware of every speech movement, to be vividly aware of himself in the act of speaking, then Al Kohol could not enter him. He would have to talk voluntarily, and since stuttering seems to be largely involuntary, perhaps he could learn to resist it. With the help of Allah!

Unfortunately, our first attempts failed miserably. Al Kohol was not to be overcome so easily. The moment Abdul entered a feared situation or attempted a feared word, the stuttering seizures appeared. We, Allah and I, wrestled hard for Abdul's Arabian soul, but Al Kohol always won. Finally, Abdul himself provided the clue that led to his final recovery. "It's like this," he confided. "My trouble is that I call on Allah to enter me only in these moments of threat, and then, alas, he may be elsewhere." "All right," I said, "let's get Allah in you always. From now on, you and I will start training ourselves never to make an automatic movement. Everything we do must be highly conscious. As I suck on my pipe, I shall suck voluntarily, not automat-ically. As I blow out the smoke, I shall blow it out with forceful intent. If I scratch my head, I shall scratch it strongly and deliberately. We shall live at a peak of volitional consciousness, of dynamic self-awareness. For three days we shall do this in all non-verbal activity. And we will speak as consciously as we move. We will invite Allah to inhabit our skins, not just when we are in jeopardy, but always."

No one who has not undertaken such a task can realize the amount of vigilance that living voluntarily requires. Both of us became exhausted after half an hour, but then we read the Koran and prayed as we rested. We ate voluntarily, chewed with intense deliberation. We walked that way. Every nod was a strong one, never casual. Every gesture was purposive; every posture was sensed with extreme vividness.

And what happened? Both of us felt we had grown ten feet taller. By the end of the first morning's training, I sensed a power such as I have never experienced before or since. Omnipotence! I have never been so alert, so vividly aware of personal strength. Abdul gave similar testimony and he said this without a trace of stuttering. "Allah is in me! Allah is in me! I feel him. I am not afraid. I can speak." There are always certain crucial experiences in any therapeutic process that alter lives. This certainly was one of them for Abdul . . . and in a way for me. I have never forgotten that tremendous exaltation and sense of power achieved by training myself in self-awareness and purposiveness. I have since called upon it occasionally and it has never failed me. In a way I fear it. It is awesome to be drunk with power, to feel the god-stuff in one's own human clay. A few of my friends have been induced to experiment with themselves in the same way and some of them report identical experiences; others do not. Perhaps I am more comfortable with Al Kohol as a skin-partner rather than Allah, having always considered myself as small potatoes and few in a hill, and having been over-fond of my human frailties.

But what of Abdul? He did not share my misgivings. A remarkable metamorphosis occurred. From that time onward, he worked hard and long and successfully in the conquest of his stuttering. From the furtive, suspicious, stuttering cocoon there emerged a tremendous man—strong, confident, outgoing—who has since done great deeds. I have been amazed to view his achievements. And thankful for helping me grow!

Sharing Many Lives

Another of the rewards which this profession brings is the enrichment resulting from sharing the lives of others, from living not one life but many. Like all experienced workers in our field, I have vicariously participated in the daily activities, problems, defeats and triumphs of people from many walks of life. I have played father confessor to priests and renegades. I even know something of what it is like to be an old lady with Parkinson's disease or how it might feel to be a murderer. I have seen the circus of life through the eyes of a young child. My clients (as will yours someday) have shared with me their hopes and dreams as well as their miseries. All this vicarious experience has enriched my life beyond all expectation or deserving. There are many interesting tales which clients have told me about their private lives, but since these would comprise a book in itself, I will include only one of them. The author, Henry Le Grande, a stutterer from Uruguay, has given me permission to recount it here in his own words.

Every summer, we used to go to a little beach town called La Paloma (The Pigeon). One day our maid told my mother she knew a *curandero* (shaman, or witch doctor) who was infallible and who could cure my stuttering. My mother didn't believe in those things, but "Who knows?" she said. Therefore, to the shaman went I and my mother, after promising her not to tell my father because "If your father knows it he'll kill both of us."

The curandero looked and looked at me very much concentrated with piercing black eyes. Then he told my mother, "Please let me alone with him." I was frightened. For five minutes he was silent, then he started to make me embarrassing questions: Did I ever masturbate? With which frequency? Did I go to bed with the maid? To this last question, by the face he made when I told him, "No way. She is too fat and ugly," I thought he probably had some intimate relations with her.

After this briefing my mother was called back, and the shaman said that her son still had some hope of losing his stuttering. Then I was sent outside and my mother started bargaining the fee. Pretending principle, he refused to charge anything. But my mother was told by the maid that she should "donate" some chickens to the shaman. He refused them at first. How will he dare to charge to the daughter and the grandson of the famous doctor? No way. My mother insisted, and his resistance started to be weaker when he realized that my mother had really started to believe in his sorcery and beliefs.

Wives in my country are very stingy. My mother started by offering 2 chickens (was she tight!). His face was like stone. Three, four, five, six, she went up—and up, and up, up to fourteen chickens. He smiled. The deal was made. But in an explosion of motherly love, she even topped it off with this: "If my child is cured I will give you a bottle of cana and another of grappa." My mother was sure now that all power and might were with me, that I would be cured.

The shaman told us the first step would be a "purification." To achieve it, I would have to stop masturbating or even touching girls while dancing for two weeks. I would have to attend mass and confess and comulgate every day for two weeks. This was a real problem because our beach town, La Paloma, had the visit of a priest from the nearest city only on Sunday. Therefore, I would have to pedal my way out of my stuttering. During two weeks, except on Sundays, I would have to start bicycling to Rocha, a city 28 miles away.

At this time, you should know that the Catholic church was very severe and the Holy Communion was allowed only if during the twelve preceding hours no food had been swallowed. So there I was bicycling 28 miles, starting at night at 4 a.m. with a flashlight so weak that many times the moonlight was stronger. With no food and rumbling stomach too. Lord, that's motivation. Besides no dance or anything else during 14 days!! But I wanted cure for stuttering bad.

The route was hilly and dirty, and full of rocks. Dangerous! Sometimes when I let the bike coast downhill I caught a glance of a huge stone missed by inches. This reassured me that God was on my side. Also, every morning I had to urinate in a bottle of Coca Cola and my mother should take it to the curandero. It was important. After the purification stage passed, he called my mother and told her that after examination of my "waters" he arrived to the conclusion that "somebody" had made the "damage" and had put the curse of stuttering on me. She was to provide a picture of that person.

My mother thought and thought, and finally remembered that when I was four or five years old, a maid used to put a paper sack on her head and scare me half to death. Ah, that was the one!!! But where to get the picture? It was impossible to trace her down after so many years. It was a dead end. My mother was desolate. The curandero suddenly must have realized that the promised chickens were getting far away. So after one full day of meditation he found the solution. My mother must bring the picture of any woman my mother really hated. Then he would act, and my stuttering would be passed on to this hated woman and I would be free of the curse and talk free. He also said that I should have to learn by heart a kind of incantation poem in a language he said was Quechua, an Indian tribe from the Andes Mountains, whose first words were, as I remember: "Bororo, Bororo, Bororo, cu ma cha ua, cu ma cha ua." And so I did. I said it a thousand times. "Bororo, Bororo, Bororo, cu ma cha ua, cu ma cha ua."

Since my mother didn't have any enemy, she had a real problem finding the necessary picture. Suddenly, in an inspirational moment, and with a sadistic grin, she said, "This will teach her," and she found a picture of Eva Peron, the wife of the Argentinian dictator, who they said had been a woman of dubious behavior before her husband was elected president of Argentina. My mother disliked Eva Peron. According to her, no decent woman in South America could approve that kind of First Lady. The purpose was clear. My stuttering would go to Eva Peron. What a revenge for decency and good behavior, thought my mother.

At last all was ready, but two things were bothering me: (1) during my second week of purification my stomach and hunger had gotten more strong than my motivation and I had sneaked out some pieces of bread in my pockets before leaving the house for my long bicycle ride; (2) I also started to think what if Mrs. Peron had a very good curandero at hand. After he examined her "waters" would he discover who had done the "damage"? And would he get back at me?

Next step was to wait for a night with full moon and a halo around it. I waited. Then one night I was awakened by my mother. The maid was waiting for me outside in the dark. I followed her up to the village where the curandero was waiting for me. "Follow me," he commanded. I followed him across the fields up to a little shack. Inside there were three or four candles and a little glass. Then I had to drink a mystery liquid that tasted terrible and then go out to look at the moon and start to say very slowly and loud the incantation.

I started: "Bororo, bororo, bororo, cu ma cha ua, cu ma cha ua." This I repeated many, many times and without stuttering one single time. I was surprised, shocked. I looked at the man and for the first time I saw in his eyes under the dim light of the candles, a spark of emotion and ecstasy. I think he was really shocked and surprised that his hocus pocus had worked. I ran fast to my house. My mother was waiting. I talked, and talked, and cried, and talked. My sister got up. I continued talking. I was afraid of stopping and being unable to start again.

During one week, I was in Heaven. Full of false fluency. Full of joy. Then it happened. Somebody made the remark that I was not stuttering anymore. Next day I was stuttering bad as ever. The curandero was surprised. After two days of "consultation" he started asking me questions. What went bad? I knew, but I never confessed that I took the bread in my pocket and ate it when I made the long bicycle trip and this probably weakened the power of the whole thing. No, I never told him. So he arrived to the conclusion that Mrs. Peron must have a very powerful curandero. A stronger shaman than he. The might of being in power. Or in his own words, "There much, much money there." My curandero's magic was not strong enough.

Many years later another maid, Dona Jacinta, took me to her own curandero. When I told him my first experience, and especially when he heard the man had pounded nails in the mouth of Mrs. Peron's picture, he whistled, looked at the ceiling in astonishment, and told me, "This guy was really using hot stuff!" I was then a little more convinced that it was the bread I ate during the purification stage that weakened the whole thing.

Somehow I had avoided an international crisis but it was hard to find stuttering nails in my mouth again forever.

Speech pathology is a fascinating profession. One is often frustrated but rarely bored. Day after day, to be in the front row of life's theater, closely identifying with some actor as he plays or replays his tragic or comic roles, has been both exhilarating and cathartic. But in this profession we are not merely spectators of the human drama; we have to go on stage, too, since our clients cast us in a hundred roles as they work out their personal conflicts. They have viewed me as the villain, the devoted friend, the cruel father, the nurturing mother, the monster—yes, even the unwilling lover at times. Under the cover of the clinician-client relationship lies a theater—sometimes the theater of the absurd.

Some of my most interesting and challenging clients have come from the church—priests or preachers or seminarians. Most of these men of the cloth either stuttered or had voice problems, mainly the latter. Fortunately, styles of preaching have changed over the last four decades, but in the early years of my practice sermons had to be full of fervor, vocal strain, hell and damnation if the preachers were to be judged as effective or sincere. Often they used a strained throaty voice quality, "the preacher's voice," lugubrious in its tones of doomsday as they loudly exhorted their sinners to seek salvation. You must remember, too, that then there were no microphones or amplifying sound systems. As a result, vocal nodules and contact ulcers from the vocal abuse were so prevalent that both were included under the commonly used diagnostic label, "clergyman's throat."

I always dreaded the holidays of Christmas and Easter, for I knew that soon some minister would be coming to the clinic because his voice had broken under the strain. Not that they were so difficult to help, for most of them improved rapidly after surgery, rest, or a program of vocal hygiene, but I knew I would have to listen to their sermons and prayers as they practiced speaking without straining. And I guess I never really learned to handle their attempts to save my soul. When they found I did not go to church, each one was bound to convert me. One even tried to make me into a Mormon, a Latter-day Saint. To help a client change, some identification on the part of the clinician must take place and I've always had trouble identifying with preachers or priests.

Occasionally I found myself in the role of father confessor, listening to strange and wondrous tales of temptation and big and little sins. And there have been times when I've dispensed my own brand of absolution or even suggested appropriate ways of paying penance when the hysterical aphonia was clearly the consequence of too much guilt. Many of these men were very much alone and what they needed most was a trusted person in whom to confide their human frailty. I shall not reveal the secrets with which they honored me.

But I can tell you about George, a Baptist preacher from Alabama. He was one of those stutterers who can speak very well when playing a role. Perhaps you have heard of actors who were completely fluent on stage and yet who stuttered severely in all ordinary communication. George was basically such an actor and he had deliberately entered the ministry to solve his speech problem. "God doesn't stutter," he told me, "and as a man of God, I didn't either." When he spoke with the voice of God, very throatily, he didn't stutter, and he spoke that way all the time, even when ordering ham and eggs.

After his ordination George became the minister of a small congregation in a little Alabama town. He was very well-liked and all the church members felt that he was the best preacher they had ever had. Unfortunately, his sense of fraudulence grew with each passing month, and the anxiety that his stuttering might break through his pious facade increased every Sunday. Then it happened. George was to conduct the baptismal ceremony for the son of the most important member of his congregation, Deacon Schmidt.

Quite a gathering came to witness. George cleared his throat, successfully intoned the first part of the ceremony, but when he came to the word "baptize" he knew he could not possibly say it without stuttering severely. He stopped and tried again, "I... bb...." He changed the intended word to "christen" but couldn't say that either, then back to "baptize" and back again. What other word could he substitute? The time pressure flared and the Deacon and the others looked at him waiting and wondering at the long pause. George panicked. "I... I... bb... chr... I dunk thee in the name of the Lord!" he cried, and with that utterance he bolted from behind the altar and fled down the aisle and out of the church, never to return.

After therapy with us George became the best paint salesman for Sears Roebuck our local store had ever employed. Yes, sometimes our theater is the theater of the absurd.

Appreciation

Low on the list of rewards that a career in speech pathology has given are the thanks and appreciation received for the work done. Somehow I have always felt embarrassed when clients verbalize their gratitude and only rarely have I been able to handle such situations with any grace. Perhaps there is still some personal insecurity which makes me prefer to give rather than to receive. Perhaps, by giving, I establish potlatch claims on those who receive my services. But neither of these explanations rings the silent gong of truth that reverberates in my skull when I am dishonest with myself. Instead it is rather that I feel *I* am the one who should do the thanking, not the client. It is he who has enriched me, helped me grow and made my life meaningful. Though I have been the necessary catalyst, the solution existed within the client. I keep remembering what Michelangelo said to the bystander who asked him how he could carve those marvelous angels out of a block of marble. "Oh," said the sculptor, "they are already in that marble. All I do is chip away the stone that surrounds them." Finally, I always have a keen sense of my own limitations as a therapist. Hundreds of forces, both past and present, bombard my client. I am only one of many. To feel that I alone have been responsible for his change seems both unrealistic and egotistic. The following bit of personal history may illustrate my attitude toward appreciation.

I think I was first hired because the President of our university had a wife whose favorite nephew stuttered badly and who had been unable to get any relief from the quacks who preyed upon stutterers at that time. Indeed, he had gone to one of the same stuttering institutes that I had attended—one where we were taught to swing our arms in a wide arc as we uttered each syllable. Once we had mastered that, we were told merely to pinch our forefinger against our thumb to time the moment of speech attempt. When we went downtown, we kept our hands in our pockets and did the pinching therein. It looked a bit indecent, but initially the distraction did seem to help, though the speech seemed strange and labored. Unfortunately, as soon as the trick became habitual it no longer distracted us from our fears and the stuttering returned. I even found I was stuttering with my fingers—that I couldn't pinch.

Anyway, I was hired to build a speech clinic, one of the first in the country. I knew a lot about stuttering but nothing about all the other speech disorders. All my training had been in psychology and I've never had a single course in my own field. I've had to learn from my clients. In the early 1930's, there were few decent books on the subject of speech pathology; very little professional literature existed. I needed information, hungered for it, for I knew I needed it to help my clients. Yet sometimes today I feel sorry for our students who have so much to read and remember—might be better for them if they could see the problems with virginal eyes rather than those clouded by too much information and misinformation.

The quarters they gave me were in an old decrepit factory building more than a hundred years old. It was dirty; the winds of winter blew right through its board siding. Rats abounded. Only fifty feet from the railroad tracks, the old dump shook and threatened to collapse every time a train went by. Whenever a parent brought in a child for an initial examination, I had to spend the first half hour trying to convince them that someone who worked in a place like that might possibly have some competency.

I was also paid very poorly, barely enough to exist—something that should be remembered in the context of the following anecdote. One day one of the rich manufacturers of our city came to me with his son, a severe stutterer. There was great hostility between them. At first the interview went poorly. They attacked each other and they attacked me. A mess! But I reflected their feelings, refused to take umbrage, tried to understand, and hunted for possible solutions. By the end of one hour, they were relaxed; by the end of two, they were interested in each other; by the end of three, a comprehensive plan of action involving both had been enthusiastically accepted. The father thanked me profusely. "You've given me back my son," he said. "How much do I owe you!" I told him there was no fee—that I was employed by the institution and that I had never charged for my services. His face grew red and he pounded on my desk furiously. "I pay for any service I receive," he shouted. "I'm no charity case. Here. . . ." and he pulled out a hundred-dollar bill, tossed it on the desk contemptuously and turned to leave. Thinking of my coal bill, long overdue, I debated silently for just a moment, then said, "I understand and accept your feelings, sir, but you should also understand mine. Observe!" And I opened the window and tossed the hundred-dollar bill out on the grass.

I'll never forgive the son of a sea cook for running around the corner of the building and grabbing it.

Despite my policy of not accepting money or gifts for services, I have had some come my way. One Christmas day, I got a call from the local Railway Express office telling me to come down to pick up the bottle of blood plasma. I protested in vain that I was a speech doctor, not a real physician, but the caller was adamant. He'd come down and opened up the damned office and I'd better hurry right down and get that plasma so he could have some Christmas, too. It had come from San Francisco, from Julius Lucoff, one of the zaniest stutterers I've ever helped. The blood plasma turned out to be a quart of Vat-69, a scotch whiskey which I had been known to imbibe anon.

Another treasure of mine is a large purple and black cod-piece, knitted by the mother of a stutterer from Nome, Alaska to help keep his testicles warm. And there are always the phone calls and letters, family snapshots and newspaper clippings of achievements from clients whose names I have almost forgotten but whose symptoms I recall very vividly. But far more important than these rewards has been the privilege of seeing human flowers that once you weeded with care and fertilized with faith and hope, come finally into bloom.

Another real boon provided by a career in speech pathology is the opportunity to learn new things. One of my students told me he couldn't wait for graduation so he could stop learning and start practicing his profession. I responded by saying that he could then stop memorizing and really start learning how to learn. Certainly this continual learning is not only necessary; it can also be exhilarating. Our field of speech pathology is in constant flux; new information and new methods for helping our clients appear every year. No one can be even halfway competent unless he keeps abreast of these changes. But you don't have to memorize a damned thing—and that too is very, very good.

When I once had a half-year sabbatical leave to roam the Caribbean and Central America, I felt I was abandoning my students. To relieve myself thereof I wrote them this:

One of the basic laws that seems to govern all living things is that they continue to grow or they begin to die. In forty years of training therapists, I have been saddened all too frequently when I observed the symptoms of rigor mortis setting in my students as soon as they graduated and began to practice their profession. I have watched their first fine enthusiasms fade, their dedication to the healing of the people they served grow faint and weaken, and their self-esteem decay. It is a sorry sight.

I have sought to discover why this tragedy occurs in some persons and not in others, for I know personally that it need not occur. At the unripe age of sixty-five I still have the conviction that I am continuing to grow. If this is only an illusion, it is hard to explain why each day brings so many new insights, new awareness and new learning, when each month provides its quota of interesting experiences, when each new year holds more promise of things and thoughts to explore. The tick-tock of time may govern the aging of the flesh but the spirit does not seem to need to plod to its tempo. In these salad years of mine, it is the antic Dance of the Wild Cucumber that provides the rhythm of my days.

Some persons collect stamps or coins or match covers. I collect people—a far less expensive and more interesting hobby, for they come in all sizes, shapes, colors and characteristics. Since each of these human beings is unique, as stamps are not, each offers the collector the opportunity for new learning and vicarious growth. I have known fairly intimately all sorts of people—priests and professors, mill-wrights and farmhands, saints and sinners, young fools and old ones. With little children I have explored the holes of the ground and with their parents the holes of the head. I have shared the goodness of sweaty labor during the harvest season and the veiled thoughts of a sad wife enslaved in her kitchen. How anyone could find himself bored in a world so full of human frailty, folly, triumph and despair is hard for me to understand. Each dawn lifts its curtain on a stage where a thousand large or small tragedies or comedies are enacted daily. Why must some of us drink of our small cup of time with eyes closed? Why do some of us need drugs to seek vivid experiences when they are all about us everywhere for the asking? Or, worse yet, why ingest other drugs to dull sensibilities that already are covered with too many buffering callouses? Better to die of a rose in aromatic pain than to sit there dully, wondering why your life, like old salt, has lost its savor.

Anyway, what I guess I am trying to say to you is that our profession offers tremendous opportunities for personal growth since it puts us in close contact with a wide variety of people. Each one of these can teach us something, can open doors to new perceptions, can stimulate our own growth if we will try to identify with them enough to let us learn something new. All of them, and especially the little children whose eyes are still able to see things afresh, can be our teachers. There is so much to learn about how to live well that we need every teacher we can get. I reject the view that we are captive laboratory rats completely controlled in the maze of our particular environment by the reinforcements and punishments of Fate, that all-knowing operant conditioner. If we can learn enough, and keep learning, we can shape our own lives enough to triumph over incredibly formidable obstacles. I have, in my collection, many people who have done so and I treasure them, for they have shown me that we are responsible for the quality of our existence. What is more, the impact they have had on me has taught me that I can have impact too, which is what life is all about if it is to have any meaning whatsoever. In our profession we are blessed by being presented with a constant opportunity to have this impact on others so that they will live better lives. Better to be a flawed but useful tool than a slowly tarnishing ornament! There's much work to do in the vineyard.

In saying these things I do not wish to imply that one always has to have a living, breathing, smelly human being as one's teacher if growth is to continue through new learning. Some of the best of my teachers have come in sizes smaller than seven by ten inches—the books and periodicals I've read. I have known students to stop reading anything but the comics in the evening newspaper as soon as they got their master's degrees, and in a way I can't blame them though I regret their deprivation. So much of our higher education requires far too much mandatory reading of the professional literature in order to get the scarlet letter A and to graduate. Cramming corn down the gullet of a goose may make it more palatable but not wiser.

In far too many courses, students read solely to find out what the author thinks rather than to think about what the author has to say. This certainly helps them pass their examinations, but it does little to encourage them to keep reading the rest of their lives. And that's too bad. My own study is filled with books from ceiling to floor (and behind the chairs, and under the table, much to the disgust of my wife, The Madam) and they range all the way from *The Anatomy of Melancholy* to *The Transparent Self* to *The Handbook of Speech Pathology* or *The History of the American Outhouse*. These, too, have been my teachers—and my friends— for I have rarely purchased a book that I have not previously read and profited from. Moreover, most of them I have re-read or browsed through many times. This browsing is important since, having lived a very busy life, I have seldom had any long free periods of time available for extended reading. Nevertheless, in every day there are always a few moments of freedom each of us can take or make which otherwise might be wasted unprofitably. So I read what I can when I can.

What is important, however, is that I read not one book at a time but two—the book the author wrote and the book of my own mind. I am not content to know only what any author has to say; I want to scrutinize the thoughts that his writings trigger in my own head. I want to feel them, taste them, chew them, put them aside and then consider them again. Some of the best (and worst) books I have ever read were these shadow commentaries of my own. At times the thoughts or feelings stimulated by my reading are trivial and of little value, yet I still consider them seriously since I know that occasionally I will discover some insight that may change my life and impact on others. Of course, books and articles vary markedly in their ability to foster this parallel commentary that accompanies reading, but one never knows in advance which ones will do so. Even some of the most miserably written articles in our own professional journals have stimulated some excellent self-talk once I had wrestled my way through them, cursing every opaque paragraph.

However, I certainly do not confine my search for new significant ideas to our professional literature, though I have perhaps read more on the disorder of stuttering (even including translations from the Bulgarian) than any man now living. Indeed, I discover golden nuggets of insight and information in the most unlikely places. Each year I explore some intellectual area in which I am woefully ignorant—and there are many of them. About seven years ago, to cite but one example, I intensively studied the baroque architecture and painting of Spain. Surprisingly, the payoff was remarkable in terms of my understanding of abnormal perception, and I have ever since been better able to empathize with the elaborately twisted, distorted thinking and feeling of many of those I serve. Not that I restricted my reading during that year to that topic, either. Indeed, I seem to require a varied reading diet to continue to generate new awareness of the riches which life offers to the hungry spirit. A smorgasbord of everything from the bawdy to the sublime is most satisfying. Soul food is always available to those who hunger. If one is to continue to grow, one must feed upon it.

As I grow older, I observe with some concern that I grow more fond of the older literature that no one of my acquaintance seems to read any more—Montaigne, Shakespeare, the Brahma-sutra, the poems of Francoise Villon, and other works. These Old Ones speak to me and turn me on much more than they did when I read them in my youth. Perhaps they do so because their very survival testifies that what they have to say is important, while much of our current fare is not. Once when I was a very young man, I tried to purchase a fine meerschaum pipe from an old tobacco merchant in Chicago and, incredibly, he refused to sell it to me. "You're too young to appreciate it," said he. "Save something for your old age." (I'll have to buy one some day!) Anyway, the Old Ones have become increasingly able to stimulate the growth of my mind and I find pleasure as well as comfort in what Chaucer had to say five hundred years ago: "For out of the olde fields, as men seyeth, cometh al this newe corn fro yere to yere, and out of olde bokes in good feythe, cometh al this newe science that men lere."

But people and books, potent as they can be in stimulating continual growth, are not enough. It is also necessary to yank the body out of the ruts and nests that it insidiously insists upon making for itself. One must seek out new experiences, explore new places, assume new roles and constantly be on guard lest he march mechanically and dully to the beat of the drummer, Death. No man should even get out of bed in the same way every day of his life. Having suddenly realized this before I arose this morning, for the sake of my hypothetical soul, I crawled out over the tailboard and grinned all the way through breakfast. Ruts, like nests, become befouled through use. We mus do new things as well as think new thoughts. And have the courage to go ovei the mountain to see what he can see. That is why, as you read this, I shall be walking along a beach on Turneffe Island, thirty miles offshore from Belize, British Honduras, hunting pirate treasure, finishing my book on the Treatment of Stuttering and trying to catch a bonefish with a flyrod. Break out of your ruts too, my friends.

Professional Growth

That is what I wrote my students. Because there are professional as well as personal ruts, I have always felt it incumbent to try out the therapy procedures offered by others in our field, to give them a fair test, and to learn as much as possible about their contributions and limitations. When this experimentation was done, I always found that I gained some valuable skills that would prove useful with certain clients, even if they were not applicable to all. In fact, because I have never found any one approach suitable to all clients, I have always tried to be a pragmatic, eclectic practitioner. I have fought being identified with any cult or school and it bothers me when others speak of Vanriperian therapy, for I have never practiced it.

In the area of stuttering, I have seen wave after wave of different theories and therapies wash against the shore of our ignorance: psychotherapy, cerebral dominance, suggestion, relaxation, semantics, and presently classical and operant conditioning. Their advocates always made great claims of success, but always, as the limitations of each approach became obvious, a new wave came over the horizon and overwhelmed it. (No one can foresee the future, but I suspect the next wave will be cybernetic in nature, and that biofeedback procedures will characterize its crest.) Fortunately, each wave brings some treasure as well as junk, and if we professional beachcombers will prowl the beaches consistently, we can always profit. The sad feature of this situation, however, is that students do not have this perspective. They find it difficult or disloyal to question the theories and procedures advocated by their instructors. They hunger for the certainties, for the absolute truths that always disappear into the sand. The open mind is uncomfortable but it is essential.

I shall relate only two of my own experimentations with all these approaches. The first deals with the use of relaxation, a standard procedure in stuttering therapy during the late 1930's, and one which has had a recent rebirth in the application of classical conditioning. Initially, I had great hopes that relaxation could solve the problem of stuttering, for most stutterers speak very well under this condition. Accordingly, I studied Dr. Jacobson's differential progressive relaxation intensively, practiced it myself, and used it with my clients. It helped some of them temporarily, and a very few of them permanently, but it became obvious that most stutterers could not remain relaxed when their fears flared, no matter how thoroughly they were trained. Then I explored the use of strong suggestion and hypnosis to induce the relaxed state, again with some success but too much failure. Yoga and autogenic therapy and Transcendental Meditation* were explored, and all of these proved valuable to me as a person and as a professional. But the kind of relaxation technique that has benefited me most came from trying to photograph a soul.

I was helping a Hindu wise man get a picture of the soul. Dr. T., the director of the department of psychopathology where I was employed, walked up to me one day and without any preliminaries said, "As of this instant, I'm relieving you of all your duties. Shackson will take care of your left-handed rats, Charles Hazzard will finish building that amplifier, and Hilden can measure the rest of those Achilles' tendon reaction times." My face fell. It was the post-Depression year, 1932, and my fifty-dollar-a-month research assistantship was all I had to live on while I struggled to complete my doctorate in psychology: fifty dollars and the carrots, lettuce, and the occasional steak I smuggled from the hospital icebox where I procured the milk for my experimental animals. I was wondering which cook had betrayed me when the director smiled. "No, you're not being fired. I just have another assignment for you—an important one. I want you to photograph the soul." He grinned evilly.

As we walked back to his laboratory in the university psychopathic hospital, he explained. A famous Hindu savant named Kima had heard of our pioneering research with brain waves and action currents. He had come to our university all the way from India because he was convinced that these electrical currents might reveal the soul in action. "I tried to tell him that these waves of electrical potential that sweep across the cortex of the brain or accompany muscular effort are physiological, not spiritual, processes," said the director, "but he won't listen. When I showed him some of our photographs of action currents he started talking nonsense about soul pictures, or something. But I've been instructed by the President of the University to show this man every courtesy, so he's all yours, son. You'll find him in the next office. Photograph his bloody soul but keep him out of my hair."

I spent most of my waking hours for three months with Kima. They were good months, for Kima was both interesting and intelligent. He mastered every shred of information about those brain waves and action currents and insisted that I do likewise so that he could discuss them with me. And then, when he found I could not understand his all-consuming hunger to find the spirit or soul, he began to teach me a bit of the strange wisdom of the East. He

*I own not one but three mantras, *Whoops* (for a depressed state), *Oom* for my normal condition, and *Tish* (for over-excitement).

insisted that I learn the seven holy postures. My knees creaked, my legs went to sleep, and my thoughts kept shifting from Karma to a girl called Katie. I sure was relieved when Kima finally evolved an experimental design.

According to Kima, the soul is active when a person is inactive but alert and attentive or imagining. So to get at its essence, all muscular activity has to cease, because that masks the soul's action. When I protested that, if this were so, the only way we could get a picture of the pure soul was to kill the subject, Kima agreed. I then suggested shyly that he ask the director to be our first experimental animal. As always, Kima made me ashamed of my irreverent levity. He patiently explained that, of course, we could not kill our experimental subjects, logical as such a procedure would seem, but that perhaps by reducing the amount of muscular activity we might be able to dimly recognize the soul's essential features. It would only be necessary to have our subjects thoroughly quiet.

So I built the apparatus. It consisted of a padded chair with arms. On one of these arms there was a narrow carriage built of wood on which the subject's arm was to be placed. This arm holder was attached near the back of the chair so that it could be swung up and down, bending the subject's arm at the elbow. Also, by means of a little motor and a rope working over some pulleys, the arm carriage could be lifted without the subject's effort. Electrodes were to be placed over the critical spots on the subject's lifting muscles so that any tiny action currents in those muscles could be detected and photographed on our oscilloscope.

The night before we began the experiment, I went over to the lab and painted the whole thing with pure white enamel. Somehow the bare wood and screws didn't quite seem appropriate for catching the human soul. I also attached a small temple gong, which Kima had given me, to the top of the contraption, so that when the arm carriage pointed straight up the gong would clang. Kima smiled when he saw it. He said that it was my essential reverence, not my irreverence, which had compelled me to make these changes.

Our laboratory was in the basement of the psychopathic hospital, right under the ward where they kept the female patients who were highly disturbed. It was not a very quiet place except at meal time, so we chose noon to give the experiment its first dry run. The procedure was as follows. After the subject was placed in the padded chair with his right arm in the carriage and the wired electrode attached over the muscles, he was to lift the arm in the carriage slowly to the vertical or gong position, then drop it. Next he was to let the arm remain passive as the motor lifted the arm till the gong sounded. Next, he was merely to *imagine* that he was lifting the arm. Then he would repeat the four steps in the reverse order. It was Kima's hope that the third and fourth steps or conditions would be the ones which would reveal the essential features of the soul in action, for these were the ones where attentive imagination alone would be present.

I had expected that Kima would desire to be the subject, but he was very firm in his refusal. "I have searched for this for forty years," he said. "I am close to my dream but it is not for me to see my own soul." So saying, he went into one of his trance-like states of meditation and I went out for a hamburger. When I returned, he hooked me up in the chair and started the cameras whirring. I raised my arm; I had my arm raised; I imagined both. I did them again in reverse order. Then Kima disengaged the camera and although I was skeptical, I felt a curious flare of excitement as we went into the darkroom to develop the film.

All the pictures looked alike! Those taken when I was imagining showed action currents not as large in amplitude, but that was the only difference. There was no profile of a soul. I made some sad joke about having lost my soul to Satan that last Homecoming night, and suggested that we try it on the director's secretary, whom I was sure had as beautiful a soul as she had legs. I also proposed that we put her leg in the carriage instead of her arm, but that was vetoed by both Kima and the young lady. So we used her arm. Again the films showed a result similar to my own. I regarded the secretary with renewed interest: perhaps she didn't have a soul either. Kima was neither amused nor discouraged. "We should not expect to see the soul so easily," he said. "I must meditate upon this thing."

The next day, his face was bright. "I now know why we failed," he said. "It is because you Americans are never still; you are never quiet. What we have found on these films is your constant tension. It has masked the features of the soul. I must teach you to be quiet so that your souls can be seen. When you have learned how to be at peace within your skin, we shall make a new recording."

So with five others, including the secretary who was getting more beautiful all along, I was chosen to learn Kima's method of relaxation. He said it was a variant of Yoga. He said he practiced it every day of his life and that that was why his face had no wrinkles in it—which was true. He told me he was fifty-four years old, yet he had the face of a ten-year-old. There in the dusty basement laboratory, Kima trained us in his relaxation. First, he sat the six of us in chairs with our right arms resting on the table. Then he told us to roll our eyeballs upward and backward—"the position of death and peace." Then, while maintaining this, we had to close our eyelids over the eyeballs and to exhale just a bit further than usual, then end the exhalation with a tiny silent sigh. Over and over again he trained us until we could follow the sequence at will. Finally he was satisfied with our performance.

"Now," said Kima, "I must tell you the last step, the heart-secret of relaxation. The eyeballs backward, the long breathe out, these are essential, but there is this also: you must come to see life as a whole. In my Yoga, the whole is the circle. In my body the circle is my navel. You must therefore also see life as a whole. Meditate upon your navel."

Not a one of us ever learned to relax the Yoga way. Everytime we thought of our navels our eyeballs went down. Kima gave up and went back to

India. Sometimes, remembering my lost youth, I ring the gong for him. Nevertheless, when I really need to relax myself or one of my clients, I use Kima's first two steps.

I have also explored the use of operant conditioning and have continued to employ it with most of my clients, though rarely as the sole approach. It is a strategy that often works wonders in strengthening or shaping newly acquired behaviors, but like all strategies it has its limitations, too. I have routinely used both mild or token punishments contingently, and the escape from unpleasantness (negative reinforcement) as agents in the unlearning and learning experiences of therapy. Often I have found that, by combining the mild punishment of old habitual responses with positive or negative reinforcement for the new desired ones, much progress can be achieved. In the following account of some group therapy, you will find this combination of classical and operant conditioning as well as the use of multiple reinforcers.

One spring I received an invitation from the director of a college speech clinic in Texas to put on an intensive workshop demonstration therapy program with eight or nine severe stutterers. A fairly large group of speech therapists would attend the all-day, two-week sessions and I would not only have to lecture to them but, more importantly, I would have to do direct therapy with those stutterers. Could I show that I could do what I had said could be done for such stutterers? I could use some of her beautiful female student clinicians to assist me in the therapy. I could have anything I wanted. Would I come? I could not resist the challenge.

I remember those two weeks as the most strenuous of my existence. For one who had been a child of Lake Superior, it was hotter than hell both day and night, almost impossible to sleep, sometimes almost impossible to breathe, though one room in the clinic was air-conditioned. The stutterers were a motley group of sad sacks, all very severe avoiders, strugglers, saboteurs, all male adults. Most had experienced public school or clinic therapy for years, had failed to improve, and had little hope. I had only ten days and a weekend to prove my competence as a clinician of stutterers.

From the scanty clinical notes of the experience I present the following reconstruction of my travail:

9:00 A.M.   This hour, each day for the two weeks, was devoted to an exposition of the nature of stuttering and the goals and methods of therapy. The stutterers, students, clinicians and visiting clinicians studied the two chapters in my text *Speech Correction* that dealt with stuttering, and my lectures were amplifications and illustrations of the material therein.

10:00 A.M.   During this hour, I held a group session with the stutterers and the student clinicians who were assigned to each of them. The stutterers sat with me about a round table with the clinicians in chairs behind and slightly to one side of the stutterers. All my interaction, however, was with the stutterers—the students were only observers. The basic aim of these sessions was to build a group unity in which the stutterers identified with me and I with them—and the student clinicians with their clients. The latter was accomplished by having them stutter in pantomime whenever their client did, and in the same fashion. Sessions were used primarily to ventilate feelings about stuttering, to recount and recall past experiences in which they had stuttered badly, to verbalize their doubts and difficulties, to present excerpts of their autobiographies verbally, to ask the questions which were troubling them. If possible, I got the stutterers to answer the questions or would do so myself, but the major role I played (and which was soon adopted by the other stutterers) was that of reflecting the feelings being expressed. I also served as a goal object—as a fluent stutterer.

11:00 A.M.   During this hour the student therapists and their clients worked individually on specific subgoals that had been described in the 9:00 session. Each stutterer would be selected in turn and worked with briefly before the entire audience (about 60 people), using the applause of the group as reinforcement for specified success. I tried always to see that each stutterer displayed some success and got that applause. These demonstrations would each last only about five minutes for each stutterer and between each there was opportunity to provide a commentary on why I had done what I did and for my evaluation of the results. Pertinent or impertinent questions from members of the audience were also answered at this time.

12:00 NOON.   The stutterers ate lunch as a group with no other person present. According to their later reports, these sessions provided an opportunity for free expressions of resistance, doubts, and self- and other confrontations. They also built unity.

1:00 P.M.   I worked briefly with each stutterer and his therapist individually, illustrating the kinds of activities and experiences desired, and stressing the behaviors to be reinforced or extinguished. During the rest of this two-hour period, the stutterer and his clinician carried out a similar kind of therapy including a recording session.

3:00 P.M.   *Swimming Pool Therapy.* Since it was very hot, we (I, the stutterers and their clinicians) drove out to the home of one of the students who had a swimming pool and we spent at least an hour in that pool. My mandate was that you could only remain in the water if you continued talking so they talked continuously, shifting freely from one of the attractive female clinicians to another in this situation. However, each clinician was to reward any instance of success by some kind of affectionate gesture (pat, embrace, etc.), and to duck the stutterer's head under water for each failure. The session ended by going into the air-conditioned house for coffee, cake and ice cream, but this was contingent upon being able to make a two-minute speech demonstrating that he could fulfill the specified requirements of the day. If the stutterer could not do so, he had to work with his clinician there in the hot sun (not in the pool) until he could be successful.

5:00 P.M.   We then drove the stutterers back to the college dormitory where they remained alone without assignments until 6:30 P.M. Then they ate together again, bellyached and cursed my therapeutic guts. I used the period to talk to the student clinicians as a group, to give them an opportunity to express their problems and difficulties in working with their cases and to redefine the goals and activities for the next day. I also sought to build a group spirit among them too, and apparently did so.

6:00 P.M.   During this period I ate a little, collapsed and worked out my program and goals for the following day.

9:00 P.M.   *Beer Bottle Therapy.* Since it was almost as hot in the evening as it was during the day, and sleep was very difficult, I added another therapy session. All of us, stutterers and clinicians, drove to another town where they had an old-fashioned German barroom with a large round table. I bought the beer for all hands but it was placed in the center of the table, on the top of which I had drawn with chalk a series of concentric circles. The stutterers had to earn each swig of beer for themselves or for their clinicians by doing a specified speech task successfully—one which I designed on the spot to fit the individual needs of each stutterer. All of us were terribly thirsty and the beer was very good. I served as the judge of success and drank my own beer with gusto continuously. However, I also set up quotas of successes which would deprive me of drinking for five minutes and, as you can imagine, they worked hard to accomplish this. Each stutterer or clinician, once his beer bottle had been progressively moved from circle to circle out to the periphery where they sat, could drink as much as he could manage before taking a breath, but then the beer bottle had to be returned to the center of the table and he had to earn the next drink for himself or his partner by another series of successes. Also, failure was punished by having the clinician push the beer bottle back one ring toward the center of the table. The tasks and criteria were always tailored to the individual stutterer's needs so that he always had more success than failures and managed to drink enough himself, or to provide it for his clinician, to keep therapy progressing. The whole experience was hilarious, the fellowship was excellent, and great progress was made. Often we barely got back to our sleeping quarters by midnight, but the tasks were programmed so that the driver never got drunk. I, at least, slept very well.

By the end of the two-week period, all the stutterers were remarkably fluent. They were not avoiding words or speaking situations but seeking them. Their contortions and struggle had disappeared. Though some of them showed a few miniatures of their former responses, most of their disfluences were so slight as to be unnoticeable. And they felt very good about themselves. I found out later that some of them experienced relapses afterwards but some retained their gains and not one of them ever became again as severe as he was at the onset of the therapy. One of them is even the director of a college speech clinic. Two weeks is a short period in which to change the *behaviors* and attitudes of a lifetime, but all of us accomplished much. So here's to operant and classical conditioning!

It should be stated, however, that most of my therapy has been based on cognitive learning theory rather than conditioning. Our human clients learn in many ways and it seemed unwise to fail to use their ability to achieve insights, to make plans, to learn vicariously, to discover the new perceptions that speed the course of therapy and profoundly alter lives. Over and over again, a single, crucial, insightful experience has enabled a client to achieve a quantum jump in progress, to produce more real change than hours or months of conditioning. Accordingly, much of my therapy—and I'm sure that of many other clinicians as well—has been structured so as to promote these crucial insights and to create the conditions that facilitate their occurrence.

Many examples of this "one trial learning" could be given, but let me tell you of a single sentence that set me free from my own wretched stuttering and changed my whole life. It was spoken by an old man in a Model T Ford who had picked me up while I was walking along a country road north of Rhinelander, Wisconsin. Only the fact that I was very tired let me accept his offer of the ride, for I knew that I would immediately be asked a lot of questions and so would have to stutter miserably. But at first the old man did all the talking, a lot of it, and though very fluent, his speech was rather jerky, with many little gaps or slightly prolonged sounds. A little odd, but very fluent! I did not really pay much attention to it until after he suddenly asked me my name and where I was going, etc. My resulting stuttering was so very severe I felt he couldn't possibly understand what I was saying, and that of course only made the blockings worse.

Suddenly the old man began to laugh uproariously, so hard he had a hard time steering. He laughed and laughed, so I was furious. I could have clubbed the old bastard. I tried to tell him or motion to him to stop so I could get out but I stuttered, badly again. And again he laughed. Finally he stopped and said, "Son, take it easy. Take it easy! I'm not laughing at you but at the craziness of it all. I'm a stutterer too. And until a few years ago I used to jump around and gag and make faces just like you. But no more! *I'm too old and too tired to stutter so hard so I stutter easy.*"

The fourteen words of that last sentence hit me like a bolt of lightning.

Theretofore I had always tried to talk without stuttering, or to struggle and jerk myself out of my blocks at the cost of great effort. And always in vain. Thoughts rushed madly through my head. "Maybe I've been taking the wrong path. Don't try *not* to stutter. Stutter easy! Learn to stutter! That old gaffer is certainly fluent even though he has more blocks than I have. Learn to stutter fluently! Damned if I'll wait till I'm old and tired like him. I'll start now!"

"I'm too old and too tired to stutter so hard, so I stutter easy." That was the insight on the road to Rhinelander that changed my own life.

SOME FINAL THOUGHTS

Perhaps the hardest of all the things a clinician must learn is how to live well. You cannot heal a person's wound if you are a dirty bandage. Unless you are a healthy, strong person, your impact will be minimal, no matter what methods you use. There have been times when I resented my clients' expectations of what I should be, but I have noticed that over the years I have become a much better man than I hoped (or desired) to be. I have found that therapy is a two-edged chisel; it shapes the therapist as well as the client.

I also learned early that I must not become so addicted to the heady wine of satisfying other people's needs that I forgot my own. I have known some therapists who sacrificed themselves and their families on the altar of therapy, who devoted every moment of every day to service or to thoughts of it, who took their client's problems to bed and breakfast. These clinicians eventually became sick and overwhelmed and lost their ability to have impact. Accordingly, I have jealously guarded the private portion of my life that lies outside the therapy room. I have set limits on my involvement. I have programmed into my daily existence opportunities for escape, for cleansing and for renewal. All of us must learn this lesson or we will contract that insidious condition the social workers call "burn-out." Symptoms of burn-out can be either apathy, anxious over-concern, the resorting to mechanical methods, rut behavior, the presence of extreme fatigue, or the loss of a sense of meaningfulness.

I am not sure that a personal account of how I managed to escape burn-out and to maintain a high level of zest for forty-five years in the practice of speech pathology will help you keep your enthusiasm too. But it might. Each of us must find our own way to remain healthy. Nevertheless, I'm sure that one essential ingredient in the prescription will be *escape*. Every contract signed by a speech pathologist should provide not only for a substantial yearly vacation but also for several daily sabbaticals, even if they last for only a minute or two, and are spent contemplating one's navel, or a mantra, or a flower, or a cloud. I have a few special tunes I can use as silent lullabies, and a mental encyclopedia of good and peaceful memories that can be opened for a moment. Also, I try to avoid any immediate shifting from one client to another without clearing my clinical computers.

Similarly, I have usually been able to protect my evenings and weekends from client invasion and to fill them with activities far removed from therapy. My hunting and fishing companions are mechanics and millwrights, not professors or other therapists. I am an organic gardener, and for years have been trying to raise The Perfect Potato. Let others seek perfection in a rose or orchid. I shall take a clod of a vegetable, as I have tried to take human clods (including myself) and turn it into a shining thing. But I raise other things too—flowers, strawberries, and a bit of hell now and then. Recently, I lost three fingers in a compost shredder, and I put the bloody compost on my sweet peas and strawberries, thereby enabling me to recycle myself while still living. Not many men have been able to smell or taste their immortality. I live in a very old brick farm house up a lilac lane, so I can do my Dance of the Wild Cucumber in the fields when the moon rides full. Freedom! I have planted ten thousand trees of every kind, and some are now forty feet tall, which means that I am too. I made my first park in a space only two feet by three in the cindery back yard of a house in the city, for I've always felt that every one should make his own park. The one on our present farm now covers several acres and it is my Ephraim, a lovely place where souls can be restored. The Earth is my mother, and I suck it like a pumpkin for the strength my work requires.

The Forest is my other parent. It has always cleansed me and I return each summer to merge with it. As a troubled youth, its deep woods and clear streams and lakes provided serenity and freedom from fear, and they still do. It is very good to be able to go back to our old log cabin there and to feel my roots, for the only perfect thing in life is a circle. Besides, I can fly-fish for brook trout and regain the patience I need so much in helping others. Also, to preserve my good memories, in a private journal at the end of a day I will try to put into words some experience that I want to recall in times of stress. Here are just two of them:

"Had a miserable and ludicrous experience this afternoon. Got a fly in my nose! A McGinnty, the yellow and black trout fly that looks like a maddened bee. I was fly-fishing for brown trout on the Pere Marquette River in a pool under a great oak tree. The only way I could get the McGinnty out to the rising fish was by making a perfect roll cast. To do this, you bring the rod up suddenly and the line comes back toward you in a circle and then arcs back into the stream. Well, this time the arc intersected with my nose and the hook buried itself deeply into the cartilage of the septum, the part that separates the nostrils. I tried to work it out with my fingers but couldn't, so I cut the leader and came back to the cabin for some pliers. The Madam laughed when she saw me, the unfeeling wench, and said something about honeycombs and flowers, but when I had her fit the pliers to the hook, she would not yank, so I had to do it. Three times I tried and my head shrieked with pain, but I couldn't budge it. So I drove in to Baldwin, a little town some miles away, and inquired about a doctor. The man at the filling station giggled and referred me to someone else who laughed and said to phone the county health nurse. When I did, she asked me what was wrong. I said that I had a fly in my nose. "Then why don't you swat it?" she replied and hung up. By this time that McGinnty was feeling about as big as a pileated woodpecker, but finally, after convulsing all the patrons of a small restaurant, I found out where the physician lived. I knocked at his door and his wife appeared. "The doctor's out fishing," she said grinningly, but she told me I could wait on the porch until he returned because by that time it was getting dark. At last the bugger came, took one look, shot some novocaine into the nose, and sliced it open. When I paid him, he said, "You damned fool. Serves you right trying to catch one of those trout on a McGinnty that big. Use a number 16 next time." I understand that the women of the Ubangi consider their husbands attractive when they wear a chickenbone in their nose.

Here is another excerpt from my private journal:

October again with the fall colors in full glory. The forest is a great stained glass window, yellow with sassafras, scarlet with maple against the green of pines among white birches. The best of seasons. This morning, weary from tramping the animal paths in the poplars after grouse, I rested on an old log among the autumn mushrooms that covered it, soaking up color against the white of winter snows soon to come. A large yellow leaf drifted down and settled on my hair and stayed there. The touch of death? My angina said yes but I said no! A golden crown had been bestowed upon me. Somehow I must have acquired merit. A bright yellow crown for an old greyhead. I wore it gloriously all the way back to the cabin.

I like to write, though for years it was agony. Then I discovered a formula that made me more productive. It has three parts: write a minimum quota of only one word a day; never stop writing without leaving the sentence unfinished; and don't look at what you have written until, like pease porridge, it is nine days cold. Though some days I write only that one word, there are others when the stuff pours off my two index fingers—always to my amazement. I revise a lot, of course, though probably not as much as I should. Anyway, this is my way of being creative and freeing myself from the world. Each of us must find some way of doing this. It is not enough to be a passive receptor; one must be a creator too.

Because I have always been rather uncoordinated, painting, sculpture,